Essential Urology in General Practice

Note

Health care practice and knowledge are constantly changing and developing as new research and treatments, changes in procedures, drugs and equipment become available.

The author and publishers have, as far as is possible, taken care to confirm that the information complies with the latest standards of practice and legislation.

Essential Urology in General Practice

Edited by
*Manit Arya, Iqbal S. Shergill, Nitika Silhi,
Philippe Grange and Simon R. J. Bott*

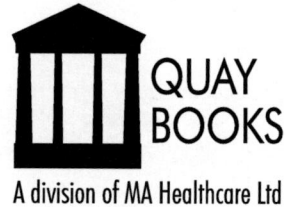

QUAY
BOOKS

A division of MA Healthcare Ltd

Quay Books Division, MA Healthcare Ltd, St Jude's Church, Dulwich Road, London
SE24 0PB

British Library Cataloguing-in-Publication Data
A catalogue record is available for this book

© MA Healthcare Limited 2009

ISBN-10: 1 85642 372 7
ISBN-13: 978 1 85642 372 4

Printed by CLE, St Ives, Cambridgeshire

Foreword

Being a General Practitioner today is a challenging profession. The GP is often presented with a variety of urological conditions, having had no or little urological experience. Many of these conditions are now dealt with in primary care – e.g. urinary tract infections, erectile dysfunction and female urinary incontinence. Unfortunately, there is no book currently available aimed primarily at GPs and trainees which satisfactorily covers this important field. Having read through this book I would like to congratulate the editors on filling this void with a simple practical text which should be essential reading to all those professionals in and related to primary care. Of particular importance is that each chapter is written as a collaboration between GPs and urologists. In these uncertain, changing times it is important to establish and maintain relationships between primary and secondary care.

I would suggest that each practice obtains a copy of this book for its library. Indeed, perhaps many hospital departments would also benefit from having a copy. In addition many GP trainees may benefit from perusing this text prior to sitting the nMRCGP.

Dr Gurdip Singh Hear
MBChB BSc(Hons) DCH DRCOG MRCGP
Principal GP Partner and GP Trainer, Crosby House Surgery, Slough
Member of the Professional Executive Committee and Primary Care
Lead, Berkshire East Primary Care Trust. Berkshire Local Medical
Committee Treasurer

Contents

Preface   ix
Editors   xiii
Contributors   xv

Part I
Adult urology

Chapter 1
Erectile dysfunction   3
Jas Kalsi, Gus Cabre, Davendra Sharma and Suks Minhas

Chapter 2
Vasectomy   15
Frank Chinegwundoh and Georgieana Cave

Chapter 3
Male infertility   25
Asif Muneer, David Jones and Suks Minhas

Chapter 4
Urinary tract infection in adults   33
Paul Erotocritou, Sima Patel, Neehar Arya, Rizwan Hamid and Petros Erotocritou

Chapter 5
Overactive bladder, urgency and stress urinary incontinence in adult females   43
Pippa Sangster, Miles Goldstraw, Rajesh Kavia, Ketan Kansagra, Vinay Kalsi and Rizwan Hamid

Chapter 6
Benign conditions of the scrotum and testis   57
Davendra Sharma, Gus Cabre and Philippe Grange

Contents

Chapter 7
Ureteric colic   **67**
Hashim Uddin Ahmed, Paul Erotocritou, Shailesh Kulkarni,
Peter Kraus and Matt Winkler

Chapter 8
Benign and malignant skin disorders of the external
genitalia   **77**
Iaisha Ali, Mohamed Hammadeh, Shailesh Kulkarni,
Navroop Shergill and Asif Muneer

Chapter 9
Lower urinary tract symptoms and benign prostatic
hyperplasia   **91**
Neil Barber and Gordon Mackay

Chapter 10
Haematuria   **101**
Aza Mohammed, Blanca Martin-Retortillo, Jay Khastgir,
Sandy Gujral and Ignacio Zamora

Chapter 11
Bladder cancer   **111**
Andrew Robinson, Azhar Khan, Iqbal Shergill, Ann McDougall and
Brian Waymont

Chapter 12
Testicular cancer   **121**
Simon Gill, Hashim Uddin Ahmed, Shashi Kumar, Manit Arya and
Jayanta Barua

Chapter 13
Prostate specific antigen (PSA)   **131**
Richard Hindley and David Love

Chapter 14
Prostate cancer – localised disease   **141**
Simon Bott, Nitika Silhi and Alison Birtle

Chapter 15
Prostate cancer – locally advanced and metastatic disease **155**
Simon Bott, Nitika Silhi and Alison Birtle

Part II
Paediatric urology

Chapter 16
The prepuce: normal development, phimosis and circumcision **167**
Nilay Patel, Vinay Kalsi, Asif Muneer, Nitika Silhi and Imran Mushtaq

Chapter 17
Urinary tract infection in children **177**
Shekhar Marathe, Jas Kalsi and Miranda Ruston

Chapter 18
Urinary incontinence in children **185**
Dawit Worku, Erdinc Havutcu, Jay Khastgir, George Fowlis and Rim El-Rifai

Chapter 19
Cryptorchidism **193**
Dawit Worku, Mohamed Hammadeh, Penelope Cox and George Fowlis

Part III
Miscellaneous

Chapter 20
Urethral catheterisation **203**
Rajesh Kavia, Vinay Kalsi, Christopher Blick, Jayanta Barua and Philippe Grange

Chapter 21
The nature and the role of the General Practitioner with a Specialist Interest (GPwSI) **213**
Nitika Silhi and Aravinda Guniyangodage

Chapter 22
Imaging techniques in urology **219**
Christopher Blick, Miles Walkden, Nilay Patel and Asif Muneer

Index **231**

Preface

Urology forms a significant proportion of primary care consultations. Most doctors and medical students have less and less exposure to this important speciality and so an easy, concise and up to date reference manual providing the essentials of urology in primary care is required.

We have produced this book for the busy General Practitioner and trainee with day-to-day practice in mind. Our aim is to promote a simple and practical approach to all urological consultations. This text will also provide an invaluable source of information and guidelines on urological management which are logical and evidence based. We hope the scope provided by this book will be useful to those sitting the nMRCGP exam. The book will additionally be of considerable interest to specialist nurses, medical students and junior doctors in related specialities.

With these goals in mind each chapter has been written by a general practitioner in conjunction with a urologist and is heavily influenced by trainee co-authors. Where possible, the chapter begins with a case study followed by suggestions for important points in the history and examination. Relevant investigations and treatment in primary care are then discussed. Further management of the condition in secondary care is mentioned in order to supplement the reader's understanding and knowledge. A list of key points can be found at the end of each section.

This book has been an exciting and challenging project. We would like to give our heartfelt thanks to all of the authors for their time and hard work. To the reader – 'Enjoy!'.

Manit Arya
Iqbal S. Shergill
Nitika Silhi
Philippe Grange
Simon R. Bott

This book is dedicated to the following:

Subhash Arya and Saroj Arya, both of whom were devoted General Practitioners and who are now enjoying retirement. They have taught me, by example, to try and live my life with dignity.

Mohan Singh and Surinder Kaur for their tireless support and sacrifices.

Ranweer and Savita Silhi for always being there. I owe it all to them.

Alan and Caroline, who have been there for me through thick and thin.

Editors

Manit Arya FRCS, FRCS(Urol)
Senior Fellow in Laparoscopic Uro-oncology, Department of Urology, Division of Surgical and Interventional Sciences, University College Hospital London, Honorary Senior Fellow in Laparoscopic Surgery, King's College Hospital, London, and Research Fellow in Molecular Uro-oncology, Prostate Cancer Research Centre, University College London.

Iqbal S. Shergill BSc (Hons) MRCS (Eng) FRCS (Urol)
Senior Specialist Registrar in Urology, St Bartholomew's and the Royal London Hospitals, London, and Research Fellow in Molecular Uro-pathology, Prostate Cancer Research Centre, University College London.

Nitika Silhi BSc (Hons) MBBS MRCGP
General Practitioner, North East London, and Clinical Assistant in Genito-Urinary Medicine, Northwick Park Hospital, Harrow.

Philippe Grange MD AIH ACCA
Consultant Urological Surgeon and Head of Section of Laparoscopic Surgery, King's College Hospital, London.

Simon R. J. Bott MD FRCS FRCS (Urol) FEBU
Senior Specialist Registrar in Urology, London.

Contributors

Hashim Uddin Ahmed MRCS (Ed) BM, BCh (Oxon) BA (Hons)
MRC Clinical Research Fellow, Department of Urology, Division of Surgical and Interventional Sciences, University College London, and Specialist Registrar Urology, Imperial College Healthcare NHS Trust, London.

Iaisha Ali MBBS MRCP
Specialist Registrar Dermatology, Churchill Hospital, Oxford.

Manit Arya FRCS FRCS (Urol)
Senior Fellow in Laparoscopic Uro-oncology, Department of Urology, Division of Surgical and Interventional Sciences, University College Hospital London, Honorary Senior Fellow in Laparoscopic Surgery, King's College Hospital, London, and Research Fellow in Molecular Uro-oncology, Prostate Cancer Research Centre, University College London.

Neehar Arya, MBBS MRCS (Eng and Ed) FFAEM
Consultant in Emergency Medicine, Canada.

Neil Barber BSc FRCS (Urol)
Consultant Urological Surgeon, Frimley Park Hospital, Surrey.

Professor Jayanta Barua, MD FRCS Ed (Urol) FEBU
Consultant Urological Surgeon and Director of Research and Development, King George Hospital, Barking/Havering/Redbridge NHS Trust, and Professor, South Bank University, London.

Alison J. Birtle MD MRCP FRCR
Honorary Clinical Senior Lecturer and Consultant Clinical Oncologist, Rosemere Cancer Centre, Royal Preston Hospital, Preston, Lancashire.

Christopher Blick MRCS
Research Fellow, Department of Urology, Churchill Hospital, Oxford.

Simon R. J. Bott MD FRCS FRCS (Urol) FEBU
Senior Specialist Registrar in Urology, London.

Sqn Ldr Gus Cabre LMS (Barc) FRCS (Eng) DRCOG DAvMed RAF
General Practitioner and Medical Officer Instructor, Royal Air Force Centre of Aviation Medicine, RAF Henlow, UK.

Georgieana Cave MBBS DRCOG MRCGP
General Practitioner, Chingford, London.

Frank Chinegwundoh MBBS MS FRCS (Eng & Ed) FRCS (Urol) FEBU
Consultant Urological Surgeon, St Bartholomew's and the Royal London NHS Trust & Newham University Hospital NHS Trust, London.

Penelope Cox MBBS MRCGP DRCOG DCH DFSRH
General Practitioner, Edgware, London.

Rim El-Rifai MD MRCPI FRCPCH DPMSA
Consultant Paediatrician and Neonatologist and Honorary Senior Lecturer in Paediatrics, Queen Mary's Hospital for Children, Epsom & St Helier University Hospitals NHS Trust, Carshalton, Surrey.

Paul Erotocritou MBBS MRCS
Senior House Officer, Urology, Whittington Hospital, London.

Petros Erotocritou MD SIM (Athens)
General Practitioner, Bramingham Park Medical Centre, Barton Hills, Luton.

George Fowlis BSc (Hons) Yale MD FEBU FRCS (Urol)
Consultant Urological Surgeon, North Middlesex University Hospital, London.

Simon Gill BSc MBBS
Senior House Officer, Imperial College Healthcare NHS Trust, London.

Miles Goldstraw BSc (Hons) MRCS
Specialist Registrar in Urology, London.

Philippe Grange MD AIH ACCA
Consultant Urological Surgeon and Head of Section of Laparoscopic Surgery, King's College Hospital, London.

Aravinda Guniyangodage MBBS MRCGP DFSRH DRCOG
General Practitioner, Brentwood, and Programme Director, King George Hospital Vocational Training Scheme, Essex.

Sandy Gujral MS FEBU FRCS (Urol)
Consultant Urological Surgeon, King George Hospital, Barking/Havering/Redbridge NHS Trust.

Rizwan Hamid FRCS FRCS (Urol)
Senior Fellow in Urology, University College Hospital, London.

Mohamed Y. Hammadeh MSc (Urol) FEBU FRCS (Eng., Urol)
Consultant Urological Surgeon, Queen Elizabeth Hospital, London.

Erdinc Havutcu MD MRCOG
General Practitioner, Palmers Green, London.

Richard G. Hindley MSc FRCS (Urol)
Consultant Urological Surgeon, Basingstoke and North Hampshire NHS Foundation Trust.

David Jones MRCP MRCGP DRCOG
General Practitioner, Witney, Oxfordshire.

Jas Kalsi BSc (Hons) MBBS (Hons) MRCS (Eng) MRCSEd FRCS (Urol)
Specialist Registrar in Urology, University College Hospital, London.

Vinay Kalsi MBBS MRCS
Specialist Registrar in Urology, The National Hospital for Neurology and Neurosurgery, Queen Square, Great Ormond Street Hospital for Sick Children, London, and University College Hospital, London.

Ketan B. Kansagra BSc MBBS DRCOG
General Practitioner, Crawley, Surrey.

Rajesh B. C. Kavia BSc (Hons) MBBS (Hons) MRCS
Specialist Registrar in Urology, Hillingdon Hospital, London.

Azhar Khan MBBS MRCS
Specialist Registrar in Urology, New Cross Hospital, Wolverhampton.

Jay Khastgir MBChB MS FRCSEd FRCS (Glas) PGCertEd FRCS (Urol)
Consultant Urological Surgeon & Senior Clinical Tutor, Morriston Hospital ABM University Hospitals Trust, Swansea

Shailesh Kulkarni MBBS MS MCh (Urol) MRCS FEBU FRCS (Urol)
Staff Grade in Urology, King George Hospital, Barking/Havering/Redbridge NHS Trust.

Shashi Kumar MBBS DRCOG
General Practitioner and GP trainer, Chingford, and Honorary Clinical Lecturer, St Bartholomew's and the Royal London Medical School.

Peter D. Kraus MBBS MRCGP
General Practitioner and GP trainer, Kingsbury, London.

David M. Love MB BS DRCOG
General Practitioner, Hook and Hartney Wintney Surgery, Hampshire.

Shekhar Marathe, FRCS MSc (Urol)
Clinical Fellow in Urology, West Hertfordshire NHS Trust

Ann McDougall MB BCh MRCGP DRCOG
General Practitioner, Elstree, Hertfordshire, and Programme Director, Northwick Park Hospital Vocational Training Scheme.

Blanca Martin-Retortillo LMS
General Practitioner, Whinfield Surgery, Darlington.

Gordon Mackay, MBChB DRCOG
General Practitioner, Crowthorne, Berkshire.

Suks Minhas MD FRCS (Urol)
Consultant Andrological Surgeon, University College Hospital, London.

Aza Mohammed MB ChB MRCS
Registrar in Urology, North Tees University Hospital, Stockton on Tees.

Asif Muneer BSc (Hons) MD FRCS (Urol)
Consultant Andrological Surgeon, University College Hospital, London.

Imran Mushtaq MBChB FRCS MD FRCS (Paed)
Consultant Paediatric Urological Surgeon, Great Ormond Street Hospital for Sick Children, London.

Nilay Patel MD MRCS
Specialist Registrar in Urology, Churchill Hospital, Oxford.

Sima S. Patel MBBS
Senior House Officer, North Middlesex University Hospital, London.

Andrew Robinson MBBS
FY2 Doctor in Urology, New Cross Hospital, Wolverhampton.

Miranda Ruston FRCS (Urol)
Consultant Urological Surgeon, West Hertfordshire NHS Trust.

Pippa Sangster BSc MRCS MSc (Urol)
Specialist Registrar in Urology, Chelsea and Westminister Hospital, London.

Davendra M. Sharma MBBCh BAO MRCS MSc FRCS (Urol)
Specialist Registrar Urology, University College Hospital, London.

Iqbal S. Shergill BSc (Hons) MRCS (Eng) FRCS (Urol)
Senior Specialist Registrar in Urology, London, and Research Fellow in Molecular Uro-pathology, Prostate Cancer Research Centre, University College London.

Navroop Shergill MBBS nMRCGP
General Practitioner, North-East London.

Nitika Silhi BSc (Hons) MBBS MRCGP
Clinical Assistant in Genito-Urinary Medicine, Northwick Park Hospital, Harrow, and General Practitioner, North-East London.

Miles Walkden MRCS FRCR
Senior Specialist Registrar, Department of Radiology, University College Hospital, London.

Brian Waymont MBChB MD FRCS
Consultant Urological Surgeon, New Cross Hospital, Wolverhampton.

Matt Winkler FRCS(Urol) MD
Consultant Urological Surgeon, Imperial College Healthcare NHS Trust, London.

Dawit Worku MD MRCS (Ed) MSc
Clinical Fellow General Surgery, North Middlesex University Hospital, London.

Ignacio Zamora LMS MD PhD
Consultant Urologic Surgeon, North Tees University Hospital, Stockton-on-Tees.

PART I

Adult urology

CHAPTER 1

Erectile dysfunction

Jas Kalsi, Gus Cabre, Davendra Sharma and Suks Minhas

Case history 1

A 65-year-old man attends his GP surgery with two-year worsening history of erectile dysfunction. Now having relationship problems. In desperation has used the Internet to order Viagra tablets. Has had no benefit. Also complaining of increasing lethargy and tiredness.

On direct questioning also complains of loss of libido and confidence. Normal examination. Morning serum testosterone is found to be low (7 nmol/l). His FSH, LH, prolactin and glucose are within normal limits. PSA 1.2. Started on testosterone replacement patches. Libido improves and erection significantly better. Adds in Viagra again; now successful intercourse.

Case history 2

Twenty-nine-year-old male. Never been able to maintain relationship as cannot get a sustained erection. No history of trauma. No long-term partner. Family worried as getting very depressed.

On direct questioning good nocturnal erections and can get success-ful erections when masturbates. Normal blood tests and examination. Referred to a psychosexual counselor and had eight sessions over four-month period. Improved confidence and starting new relationship.

Case history 3

Seventy-year-old male. Never been to see the GP before. Recently returned from Thailand after getting married to 25-year-old lady. Has had gradually worsening erections for many years and now cannot get an erection at all.

On direct questioning, no early morning or nocturnal erections any more. Gradual onset of problem. Complaining of passing urine frequently day and night. Normal examination. Fasting glucose 9.2. Fasting cholesterol 7.7; PSA 2.5; BMI 30. Waist circumference raised. Started oral hypoglycaemic agents and lipid lowering agents. Currently using Levitra successfully.

Introduction

Erectile dysfunction (ED) has been defined as the persistent inability to attain and/or maintain an erection sufficient for sexual performance.

ED is closely associated with many important physical conditions and may affect psycho-social health. As such, ED has a significant impact on the quality of life of patients and their partners. Several large epidemiological studies have shown a high prevalence and incidence of ED worldwide (see Further reading).

Increased awareness of the disease has resulted in more men seeking treatment from their GPs. Oral, intracavernosal and intraurethral pharmacological agents are now widely available in primary care. As a result, fewer patients require referral to urological surgeons, as surgical intervention has only a small specialised role in the overall management of ED.

Risk factors

Penile erection is a complex neurovascular event under hormonal control. The risk factors for ED (sedentary lifestyle, obesity, smoking, hypercholesterolemia and the metabolic syndrome) are common to the risk factors for cardiovascular disease. Furthermore, ED itself is a cardiovascular risk factor conferring a risk equivalent to a current moderate level of smoking.

History

A detailed description of the problem, including the duration of symptoms, should be obtained. Other factors that should be elicited are:

- Original precipitating factor(s)
- Predisposing factors
- Maintaining factors
- Any subsequent investigations
- Treatments, with the response achieved
- Enquiry regarding rigidity with quality of morning awakening erections, and spontaneous, masturbatory or partner-related activity erections
- Sexual desire, ejaculatory and orgasmic dysfunction
- Issues around any sexual aversion or sexual pain
- Previous erectile capacity
- Partner issues, e.g. menopause or vaginal pain
- Concurrent medical, psychiatric and surgical history
- Current relationship status and history of previous sexual partners and relationships
- Alcohol, smoking and illicit drug misuse

In the history, sudden onset of ED, presence of early morning erections and erections during masturbation/with a different partner (if has one) point to a psychological rather than organic cause of ED. The use of validated questionnaires, particularly the International Index of Erectile Function (IIEF) is advised to assess the baseline function as well as the impact of treatments and interventions.

Examination

All patients should have a focused physical examination. A genital examination is recommended, especially if there is a history of rapid onset of pain, deviation of the penis during tumescence (suggesting Peyronie's disease), the symptoms of hypogonadism or other urological symptoms. A digital rectal examination (DRE) of the prostate is recommended in the presence of genito-urinary or ejaculatory symptoms. Blood pressure, heart rate, waist circumference and weight should be measured in all patients.

Investigations

The choice of investigations depends on the individual circumstances of the patient. However, serum lipids and fasting plasma glucose should be considered in all patients.

A morning serum testosterone should be evaluated. If this is equivocal, a serum-free testosterone level should be considered. Also, if the serum testosterone level is borderline or low it should be repeated on a further morning blood sample, together with serum FSH, LH and prolactin. Discussion with, or referral to, a specialist clinic should be considered if the results are abnormal.

Serum prostate specific antigen (PSA) should be considered if clinically indicated. It should certainly be measured before commencing testosterone and at regular intervals during testosterone therapy.

Management and discussion

Coronary heart disease risk

Coronary heart disease (CHD) is associated with many of the same risk factors as ED. It is now well accepted that coronary artery disease is one end of the spectrum of generalised arteriopathy that is also likely to affect the arterial inflow to the corpora cavernosum of the penis. As the penile arteries are significantly smaller than the main coronary arteries, ED may pre-date symptomatic coronary artery disease. Many men with coronary heart disease can safely resume sexual activity and use ED therapies. However, men with unstable heart disease, a history of recent myocardial infarction (MI), poorly compensated heart failure or unstable dysrhythmia are exceptions.

Expert guidance on the management of ED in the cardiovascular patient is available (see Further reading). Patients at low cardiac risk, as defined in Figure 1.1, may be managed in primary care. Patients at intermediate cardiac risk should be re-evaluated, in primary or secondary care as appropriate, and assigned to either the low- or high-risk group. Patients that remain in the group defined as high cardiac risk should not be offerred treatment for ED in primary care. Their assessment and management should be supervised by a specialist team.

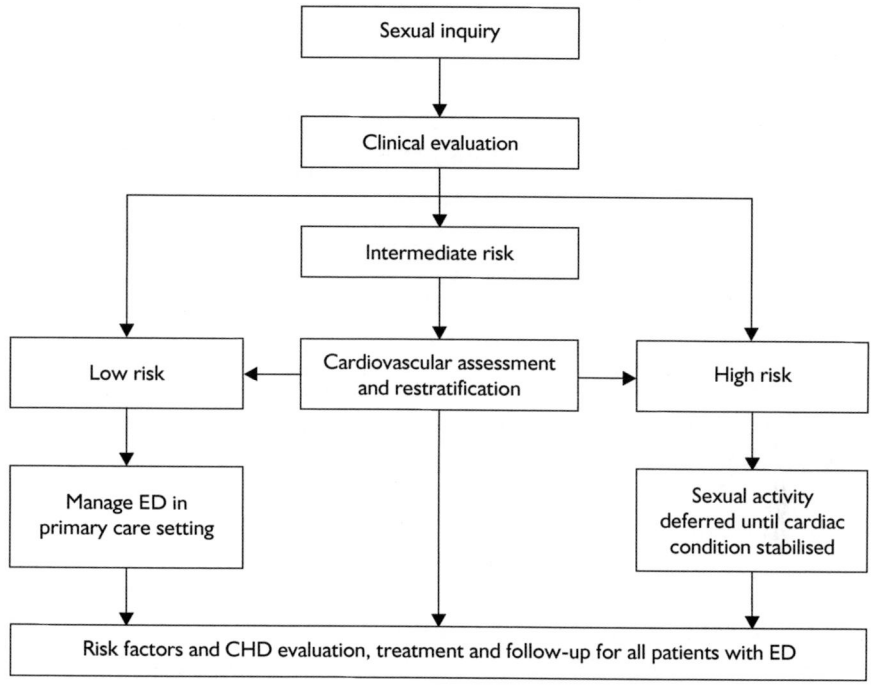

Figure 1.1 Management algorithm for cardiovascular patients.

When to refer patients for specialist investigations

Most patients do not need further investigations. However, some patients insist on knowing the aetiology of their ED and should be investigated appropriately (Table 1.1). Other indications for specialist investigations include:

- Young patients who with long history of ED
- Patients with a history of trauma
- Where an abnormality of the testes or penis is found on examination.
- Patients unresponsive to medical therapies that may desire surgical treatment for ED

Table 1.1 Specialist investigations.

- Nocturnal penile tumescence and rigidity testing
- Intracavernous injection test
- Duplex ultrasound of penile arteries
- Cavernosometry and cavernosography

Treatment

The primary goal of management of ED is to enable the individual or couple to enjoy a satisfactory sexual experience. This may involve the treatments discussed below.

Lifestyle changes

Modifications in lifestyle can greatly reduce the risk of ED and should accompany any specific pharmacotherapy or psychological therapy. Lifestyle factors include psychosocial issues, adverse side effects of non-prescription drugs and the influence of any co-morbidity. In a multicentre, randomised, open-label study, erectile function has been shown to be significantly improved in obese men with intensive exercise and weight loss versus education only. Furthermore, aggressive lipid lowering may also improve ED and may significantly enhance the effects of ED therapy in patients who are failing to respond to oral therapies.

Hormone deficiencies

Endocrine disorders such as hypogonadism, hyperthyroidism and hyperprolactinaemia may have a significant effect on sexual function. Androgen deficiency in the adult male becomes more common with increasing age; however, its management remains controversial. As well as ED, androgen deficiency is associated with osteoporosis, dyslipidaemia, Type 2 diabetes, metabolic syndrome and depression. It may also affect sexual interest, erections and responsiveness to PDE5 inhibitors. Diagnosis of androgen deficiency is based upon clinical assessment and blood testing. Men with a morning, total serum testosterone that is consistently less than 11 nmol/l may benefit from a trial of testosterone replacement therapy for ED. Hypogonadal men restored to the eugonadal state with testosterone replacement may experience a general improvement in sexual function, improved erections and enhanced responsiveness to PDE5 inhibitors. A range of well-tolerated testosterone formulations are now available, including:

- Transdermal gel (Testim®, Testogel®, Tostran®)
- Transdermal reservoir patch (Andropatch®)
- Buccal pellet (Striant®)
- Long-acting injection (3-monthly) (Nebido®)

- Traditional depot injection (3-weekly) (Sustanon®, etc.)
- Implanted pellets

Long-acting (three-monthly) testosterone injection or daily application of a transdermal testosterone gel is acceptable to most men.

Drugs and ED

A wide range of drugs have been implicated in ED. In many cases, the evidence for drugs having a direct causal relationship with some form of sexual dysfunction is relatively poor (but the patients often blame the drugs).

Psychosexual counselling

Psychosexual therapy either alone or alongside the couple's relationship therapy is indicated, particularly where the patient and or partner identify a significant psychological contribution to the problem or as perpetuating the problem.

Formal cognitive-behavioural interventions should be provided by appropriately trained and experienced therapists. They may be of some benefit in all men but are probably best used in men with a predominantly psychogenic component in ED. The concurrent use of medication, such as PDE5 inhibitors, may be more effective than using these interventions individually or consecutively.

NHS treatment

ED associated with the following medical conditions was deemed to qualify for prescription at NHS expense (which shall be endorsed SLS). The regulations do not state that these conditions must cause the ED:

- Diabetes
- Multiple sclerosis
- Parkinson's disease
- Poliomyelitis
- Prostate cancer
- Prostatectomy (including transurethral resection of the prostate: TURP)

- Radical pelvic surgery
- Renal failure treated by dialysis or transplant
- Severe pelvic injury
- Spina bifida
- Spinal cord injury
- Single gene neurological disease

There are two further qualifiers:

1. In addition, a patient qualifies if he was receiving a course of NHS drug treatment on 14 September 1998.
2. The other qualifier is if the patient is suffering 'severe distress' on account of his ED.

The decision about referral for specialist services is a matter of the clinical judgement of the GP. The Department of Health recommends referral when the GP is satisfied that the man is suffering from impotence and that this impotence is causing him (there is no mention of the partner) severe distress.

First line PDE5 inhibitors

Drugs that inhibit the enzyme PDE5 increase arterial blood flow, which leads to smooth muscle relaxation, vasodilation and penile erection. Three potent selective PDE5 inhibitors have been approved by the European Medicines Agency (EMEA) and the US Food and Drug Administration (FDA) – sildenafil (Viagra®), tadalafil (Cialis®) and vardenafil (Levitra®). These medications have proven efficacy and safety both in men with ED and also in specific sub-groups of patients (for example, men with diabetes and those who have had a prostatectomy). Sildenafil and vardenafil are relatively short-acting drugs, having a half-life of approximately 4 hours, whereas tadalafil has a significantly longer half life of 17.5 hours. PDE5 inhibitors are not initiators of erection, but require sexual stimulation in order to facilitate an erection. It is currently recommended that patients should receive eight doses of a PDE5 inhibitor with sexual stimulation at maximum dose before classifying a patient as a non-responder or failure.

Published studies on all three PDE5 inhibitors suggest that 75% of sexual attempts result in successful intercourse (i.e. the ability to maintain an erection for successful intercourse). Quoted efficacy rates are lower for patients with diabetes (55%) and after nerve-sparing radical prostatectomy (37–41%) for all three drugs. Interaction of PDE5 inhibitors and food, particularly fatty food, is greatest with sildenafil and least with tadalafil. No interaction with alcohol, up to concentrations of 0.5 to 0.6 mg/kg, has been observed with any of the three drugs.

Approximately 5% of patients do not respond to PDE5 inhibitors. Patients should be exposed to a minimum of four (preferably eight) of the highest tolerated dose of at least two drugs (taken sequentially, not concurrently) with adequate sexual stimulation. Patients should be followed up, ideally within 6 weeks of commencing therapy. So-called failure may be due to suboptimal counselling at the initial consultation, which should aim to ensure that the patient understands how to take the tablets properly and to return to the doctor if they are dissatisfied. Cost of drug therapy and reluctance of the partner are frequent reasons for unsatisfactory response.

Safety of PDE5 inhibitors and drug interactions

Organic nitrates (e.g. nitroglycerine, isosorbide mononitrate, isosorbide dinitrate), other nitrate preparations used to treat angina, such as nicorandil, and recreational drugs, such as amyl nitrate (poppers), are absolute contraindications with PDE5 inhibitors. Combined use could result in unpredictable falls in blood pressure and, potentially, catastrophic hypotension.

Co-administration of PDE5 inhibitors with antihypertensive agents may result in a small additive drop in the blood pressure, which does not usually cause significant orthostatic hypotension.

Alpha-blockers have some interaction with PDE5 inhibitors. Under some conditions, this interaction may result in orthostatic hypotension, and PDE5 inhibitors should be used with caution in patients receiving alpha-blockers.

Second line treatments

Vacuum device

See Figure 1.2: a cylinder is placed over the penis, air is pumped out with an attached pump and the resulting tumescence is maintained by a constriction ring around the base of the penis. Vacuum devices are highly effective in inducing erections regardless of the aetiology of the ED. However, the satisfaction rates may vary from 35% to 84%. Most men who are satisfied with vacuum devices continue to use them long term. Adverse effects include bruising, local pain and failure to ejaculate.

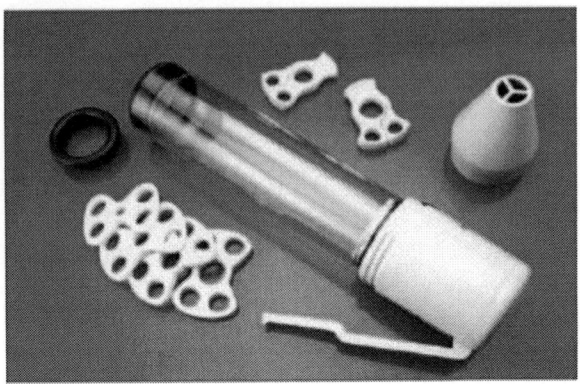

Figure 1.2 Vacuum device.

Vacuum devices are contraindicated in men with bleeding disorders or those taking anticoagulant therapy. They can be prescribed under Schedule 2 and represent a very cost-effective way of treating ED, even though initial costs are high.

Other second line treatments

These are shown in Table 1.2.

Table 1.2 Other second line treatment options for ED.

Intracavernous injection	Alprostadil (Caverject™, Viridal™)
	Papaverine (0–80 mg)
	Phentolamine (0.5 mg)
	Aviptadil (VIP) and phentolamine (Invicorp™)
Intraurethral injection	Alprostadil in a medicated pellet (MUSE™)

Specialist treatments in secondary care

Penile prosthesis

Penile prostheses insertion should be offered to all patients who fail to respond to or are unable to continue with medical therapy or external devices. It is important that patients and their partners are offered a choice of the available devices after having the opportunity to see and handle them. Penile prostheses are particularly suitable for those with severe organic ED, especially if the cause is Peyronie's disease or after priapism. New generation prostheses achieve long-term patient satisfaction and low complication rates.

Conclusions

There is now overwhelming evidence that ED is strongly associated with cardiovascular disease, such that newly presenting patients should be thoroughly evaluated for cardiovascular and endocrine risk factors, which should be managed accordingly. Furthermore, patients attending their primary care physician with chronic cardiovascular disease should be asked about erectile problems.

The availability of effective oral medication has revolutionised the treatment of ED, but not all patients are being diagnosed and treated. Oral therapies are effective in approximately 75% of patients and there is considerable evidence that adequate levels of testosterone are required for ED therapies, especially PDE5 inhibitors, to achieve maximal response. In many cases, normalisation of testosterone levels can restore erectile function. Patients who fail all medical treatments should be offered penile prosthesis insertion.

Key points

- ED is strongly associated with cardiovascular disease.
- Patients should be assessed for hypogonadism, diabetes and dislipidaemia.
- Effective oral medication has revolutionised the treatment of ED; PDE5 inhibitors should be first line treatments.
- Vacuum pumps, intra-cavernosal and intra-urethral therapies should be second line treatments.
- Patients who fail all medical treatment should be offered penile prosthesis insertion by specialists.

Further reading and bibliography

Feldman, H. A., Goldstein, I., Hatzichristou, D. G., Krane, R. J. and McKinlay, J. B. (1994) Impotence and its medical and psychosocial correlates: results of the Massachusetts Male Aging Study. *J. Urol.*, **151**, 54–61.

Jackson, G., Betteridge, J., Dean, J., Eardley, I., Hall, R., Holdright, D,, Holmes, S., Kirby, M., Riley, A. and Sever, P. (2002) A systematic approach to erectile dysfunction in the cardiovascular patient: a Consensus Statement – update 2002. *Int. J. Clin. Pract.*, **56**, 663–71.

Saltzman, E. A., Guay, A. T. and Jacobson, J. (2004) Improvement in erectile function in men with organic erectile dysfunction by correction of elevated cholesterol levels: a clinical observation. *J. Urol.*, **172**, 255–58.

Thompson, I. M., Tangen, C. M., Goodman, P. J., Probstfield, J. L., Moinpour, C. M. and Coltman, C. A. (2005) Erectile dysfunction and subsequent cardiovascular disease. *JAMA*, **294**, 2996–3002.

Traish, A. M. and Guay, A. T. (2006) Are androgens critical for penile erections in humans? Examining the clinical and preclinical evidence. *J. Sex Med.*, **3**, 382–407.

CHAPTER 2

Vasectomy

Frank Chinegwundoh and Georgieana Cave

Case history

A 45-year-old gentleman with two children and a long-term partner attends the practice requesting a vasectomy.

Introduction

The vas deferens was named by Berengarius of Carpi (1470–1530) from the Latin for 'vessel', and the Latin *'deferre'* – to carry down. Vasectomy as a deliberate procedure has been around for over 100 years. It was thought at the start of the 20th century that the procedure 'rejuvenated' men. Indeed both Freud and Yeats are said to have had vasectomies for this reason. It was also used as a means of eugenics in particular to stop 'defectives' procreating. In the 1930s onwards it found popularity as a means of preventing post-prostatectomy epididymitis, until the advent of antibiotics. It was really from the 1960s that vasectomy caught on as a means of mass sterilisation. It was enthusiastically adopted by agencies in China and India to control the birth rate. It is now a common sterilisation technique worldwide.

History

A full medical history should be taken, as for any other consultation. Enquiry should be made about bleeding disorders or co-morbidities, as that may determine the choice of anaesthesia. In particular, the patient should be asked the reason for a vasectomy and why now. It is not necessary in English law for the spouse to have to give their consent, but it is prudent to enquire if this is a joint decision. The man is asked if he is certain that he does not want any more children. It is surprising how often men have not thought things through or think that the operation is easily reversed! If a patient enquires about sperm banking ('just in case') it is usually due to uncertainty. Many hospitals and clinics offer sperm banking on a commercial basis. The costs involved with storage and *in vitro* fertilisation (IVF) at a later date are high, and successful IVF is not guaranteed.

The man is asked to think about what would happen if there were a family tragedy resulting in the loss of a child, or to contemplate his relationship ending and finding himself with a new partner. Despite this counselling, approximately 10% of men later seek reversal of vasectomy.

Enquiry is made about the number of children already and any expected and their ages. How long has that relationship been and are there children from previous relationships? What is the motivation for seeking a vasectomy? Often men will volunteer that their partner has a difficulty with contraception or that future pregnancy would be hazardous to her health. Men may say that they feel it is their turn to do something and that male sterilisation is easier than female.

Examination

On examination of the scrotum, the vasa are palpated and how easily they are located is noted. The testes are examined to exclude any abnormality such as a tumour (very rare), but importantly to be aware of conditions that may hamper surgery or dictate the type of analgesia. For example, a varicocoele may make palpation of the vas difficult, as may the presence of a large hydrocoele. In such situations my preference would be for general anaesthesia, whereby the scrotum can be explored if necessary. At times, the patient is unaware of an abnormality and may erroneously think that something untoward occurred during surgery.

Investigation

If performed using local anaesthesia no investigations are necessary. However, prior to a general anaesthetic routine pre-operative assessment and investigations are advocated.

Management and discussion

Counselling

This is very important as inadequate counselling is the main reason for medico-legal problems post vasectomy.

Men should be reassured that the vasectomy will not adversely affect their libido or erections.

The patient is counselled that he should view a vasectomy as a permanent sterilisation. The procedure should be regarded as irreversible, as successful reversal of vasectomy cannot be guaranteed, especially the longer the interval between the vasectomy and request for its reversal. In addition, whilst many health economies will pay for vasectomy, they almost certainly will not pay for its reversal. Reversal of vasectomy in the private sector is an expensive procedure with variable results. There is the option of freezing sperm, at the same time as reversal of vasectomy, for later use employing alternative techniques for conception.

If he has doubts about this choice of sterilisation, the patient should share his concerns with his primary care doctor, and perhaps reconsider vasectomy as a birth control option.

It is crucial that the man understands that he is not sterile immediately after the vasectomy. It is estimated that it takes an average of 16–20 ejaculations before the sperm stored downstream of the 'cut' are cleared. We instruct the patient to undergo semen analyses at prescribed times (usually 12 weeks and 14 weeks post vasectomy), following which we will inform them of their sterility status.

The literature quotes a 1 in 2,000 recanalisation rate, that is the 'tubes rejoining' and pregnancy resulting, even where there was previously documented post vasectomy azoospermia. Vasectomy is not a 100% 'pregnancy can never result' procedure.

The counselling also must mention the incidence of chronic scrotal pain that can occur post vasectomy. We quote a 6–16% incidence, although estimates vary. The scrotal pain can persist sufficiently for long-term analgesia to be required. In very rare cases the vasectomy is reversed to alleviate the pain. The aetiology of post-vasectomy chronic pain is uncertain. It is often envisaged to be due to sperm abutting against the tied end of the vas.

Most procedures in the UK and indeed worldwide are conducted with local anaesthesia. It is well tolerated by most. It has the advantage of safety and low cost, especially where anaesthetists do not abound.

We recommend general anaesthesia where the man is very anxious or where the man specifically expresses a preference to be 'asleep'. Scrotal abnormalities that may impede vasectomy are better dealt with under general anaesthesia. There are men in whom, by dint of their body habitus and scrotal dimensions, it is difficult to palpate their vasa. We would advise general anaesthesia in these instances. It is less stressful for the patient and the surgeon and the theatre staff.

Written information is given to the patient reiterating the counselling and a consent form signed at some stage prior to surgery.

The vasectomy takes 10–20 minutes to perform. We would advocate the availability of diathermy equipment in case of bleeding from blood vessels running alongside the vas. Cauterisation of such vessels lessens the risk of post-operative scrotal haematoma.

Operative technique

Conventional incisional technique

This is the method that is most familiar to UK practitioners. Traction downwards is applied to the testis with one hand whilst the other mobilises the vas to a superficial position just beneath the skin. The vas is fixed between two fingers and a thumb. If local anaesthesia is to be employed the skin and vas and perivasal tissues are infiltrated (1 or 2% lidocaine). A small skin incision is made over the vas. The vas is grasped with specially designed vasectomy ring forceps and delivered. It is our practice to excise a 2 cm length of vas, cauterise the ends and then doubly ligate the cut ends with 2-0 vicryl. Haemostasis is secured and the wound closed with 3-0 vicryl rapide. The wound is dressed with paraffin gauze and blue gauze and held in place by a snug-fitting athletic supporter or elasticated underwear.

No-scalpel vasectomy

This technique was popularised in China. When the vas has been fixed underneath the skin a sharp pointed mosquito haemostat is used to puncture the scrotal skin, vasal sheath, vas wall and into the lumen. The procedure proceeds as above once the vas has been delivered. This technique results in fewer haematomas and infections and just leaves a puncture wound that does not require suturing. However, it takes longer training, as technically it is more challenging.

Cut ends – vasal occlusion techniques

There are several ways of dealing with the resulting patent cut ends of the vas. Suture ligation remains the most commonly practised method worldwide. However, it is recognised that necrosis and sloughing may occur where the ligature is applied and therefore occlusion may not occur. It is our practice to excise a 2 cm length of vas, cauterise the ends and then doubly ligate the cut ends with 2-0 vicryl. To our knowledge we have not had any recanalisations and ensuing pregnancy.

Some practitioners singly ligate the ends, with either an absorbable or non-absorbable suture material. Other surgeons ligate the ends and also interpose a fascial tissue layer between them. Some cauterise the ends and do nothing further. Some workers apply one or two medium hemoclips to the vasa. Some perform intraluminal cautery and apply hemoclips. The wider diameter of hemoclips, compared with suture ligation, more evenly spreads the pressure on the vasal wall, resulting in less necrosis and sloughing. The power of the electrocautery should be sufficient to destroy a length of mucosa, but not high enough to cause necrosis of the vasal wall.

Excising a length of vas, intraluminal cautery followed by double ligation (or hemoclips) reduces recanalisation to less than 0.5%.

A single (testicular) end being 'open' gives rise to a sperm granuloma. If both vasal ends are not fully sealed (open-ended vasectomy) recanalisation may occur. The incidence of vasectomy failure ranges from 1–5% if single suture ligation is employed.

The length of excised vas correlates with vasectomy failure: the longer the length removed, the smaller the risk of failure due to recanalisation. A study by Kaplan and Huether (1975) into failed vasectomy found that the length of excised vas deferens is crucial. Less than 15 mm had up to a 25-fold greater incidence of failure.

Most urologists remove a section of vas and send it to a pathologist to verify that the correct procedure has been carried out. This is primarily for medico-legal reasons.

Post-operatively

The patient is discharged after a period of recovery. This is a walk in, walk out day surgery procedure. Scrotal support or tight supporting underwear is of benefit to reduce scrotal swelling. We would advise two weeks' support.

Return to work is rapid – a day or two later if to a clerical job and perhaps a week later if a heavy manual job.

Where absorbable skin sutures are used (we use 3-0 vicryl rapide) the man is advised that the stitches will fall out by three weeks.

Post-operative semen analysis

There is no absolute standard of care as to when to declare a man sterile after a vasectomy. Commonly, semen analysis is sought at 12 and 14 weeks post procedure. On confirmation of azoospermia the patient may be declared sterile. He is reminded nonetheless that late recanalisation can occur.

Where there are motile sperm found in the ejaculate three months post operation, it is recommended that the vasectomy is repeated.

At times there are non-motile sperm on semenalyses. Research indicates that subsequent ejaculates will become azoospermic. The man is therefore given a conditional or sterile 'clearance'. The chances of pregnancy are very low indeed, so most men do not wish to continue providing sperm samples.

Complications of vasectomy

The experience of the vasectomist is the single most important factor relating to complications.

Haematoma and infection

Haematoma is the most common complication of vasectomy. We quote a 2% incidence. We feel that the availability of diathermy during the operation allows the coagulation of vasal blood vessels and lessens the risk of bleeding and haematoma. A haematoma provides a rich culture medium for micro-organisms.

Sperm granuloma

These are formed when sperm leaks from the testicular end of the vas post operatively. The sperm cause an intense inflammatory reaction which results in a firm palpable swelling. They are usually asymptomatic.

Recanalisation

This was discussed above.

Epididymis

The brunt of pressure induced damage after vasectomy is borne by the epididymis and efferent ductules of the testis. This is to be expected, as the vas has been occluded. These structures become very distended and then adapt to reabsorb large volumes of testicular fluid and sperm products. Where pain post vasectomy is confined to the epididymis, an epididymectomy is curative in 90% of cases. On one survey, 87% of those undergoing epididymectomy had excellent initial symptomatic benefit. At 3–8 years afterward, 90% of patients interviewed had a sustained improvement of their scrotal pain. Post-epididymectomy pathological analysis revealed features of long-standing obstruction and fibrosis which may have accounted for the pain. However, epididymectomy is often seen as a 'last resort' after reversal has been tried and failed. Interestingly, the back pressure is not transmitted to the seminiferous tubules, which is why the testes can demonstrate normal spermatogenesis as long as 15 years post vasectomy.

Post-vasectomy pain syndrome or orchalgia

The incidence of chronic scrotal pain post vasectomy is uncertain. We quote up to 16% to our patients. This is pain persisting months or even years after the vasectomy. For the majority, prolonged analgesics are required. Other options include the following:

- *Spermatic cord denervation*
In general, most surveys reports that over 76% reported complete relief of pain at their first follow-up visit and were discharged. The rest of the patients had a significant improvement in the symptom score and were satisfied with the results. One survey in the journals section quotes 97% success rate.

- *Epididymectomy*
This was discussed above.

- *Reversal of vasectomy*
At times, just cutting the occluded testicular vasal end of the vas and allowing sperm to leak out, causing a sperm granuloma, relieves the pressure and the pain subsides. It is reported that 75% of patients who undergo vasectomy

reversal for post-vasectomy pain syndrome have relief of symptoms after the initial procedure. Another 18.75% may need a second reversal procedure, with half of these subsequently having relief of symptoms. Overall, 85% of men ultimately have resolution of the pain.

Antisperm antibodies

Vasectomy disrupts the blood–testis barrier, resulting in detectable levels of serum antisperm antibodies in 60–80% of men. It has been postulated that such antibodies are a factor in the failure of reversal of vasectomy when the vas is patent. However, the vogue of treating with steroids has fallen out of favour due to side effects. There is no increased risk of lupus or scleroderma or rheumatoid arthritis.

Prostate cancer

There has been controversy as to whether a vasectomy confers an increased risk of developing prostate cancer. There have been observational studies and large-scale cohort studies. A USA National Institute of Health panel concluded that the epidemiologic association between prostate cancer and vasectomy is weak and that screening for prostate cancer should not be any different for men who have had a vasectomy.

Key points

- Prior to proceeding to vasectomy the patient should be counselled that it should be considered an irreversible procedure; there is a late failure rate of 1 in 2,000 due to recanalisation; there is need for contraception until the patient provides two semen samples at 12 and 14 weeks post-vasectomy, which confirm azoospermia; post-vasectomy chronic scrotal pain may occur in up to 16% of patients.
- The majority of vasectomies are performed using local anaesthesia except in cases of undue patient anxiety, patient preference, difficulty palpating the vas deferens due to body habitus or scrotal abnormalities, when the procedure requires general anaesthesia.

- There are two operative techniques available in performing vasectomy – the conventional incisional procedure and the no-scalpel technique. The latter results in fewer haematomas and infections and just leaves a puncture wound that does not require suturing. However, it takes longer training, as technically it is more challenging.
- The experience of the vasectomist is the single most important factor relating to the incidence of post-operative complications.

Further reading and bibliography

http://www.vasectomy-information.com/index.asp. Accessed June 2008.

Kaplan, K. A. and Huether, C. A. (1975) A clinical study of vasectomy failure and recanalization. *J. Urol.*, **113**, 71–4.

Sandlow, J. I., Winfield, H. N. and Goldstein, M. (2007). Surgery of the scrotum and seminal vesicles. In: *Campbell-Walsh Urology*, 9th edn (eds. A. J. Wein, L. R. Kavoussi, A. C. Novick, A. W. Partin and C. A. Peters), pp. 1098–103. Saunders Elsevier, Philadelphia, PA.

CHAPTER 3

Male infertility

Asif Muneer, David Jones and Suks Minhas

Case history

A couple in their early 30s have been trying to conceive for the past two years without success. She has had no previous pregnancies and her periods are regular. Her FSH, LH and day-21 progesterone are normal. His only past medical history was an orchidopexy as a child and on examination both testes are of a good volume with a unilateral varicocoele. A semen analysis was arranged which revealed azoospermia.

Introduction

Infertility is defined as a failure to conceive following 12 months of unprotected intercourse.

Approximately 10% of couples are unable to conceive. Of these 20% are exclusively due to male factors and 30% are a combination of male and female factors. Therefore a complete evaluation of the male partner is essential in order to identify those males who can undergo surgical intervention.

History

Preferably the consultation with the general practitioner (GP) should involve both partners. Prior to evaluating the male patient the age of the female partner

Table 3.1 Common causes of obstructive azoospermia.

Epididymal obstruction	Post-infective (epididymitis)
	Post-surgical (removal of epididymal cysts)
	Idiopathic epididymal obstruction
Vas deferens obstruction	Post-vasectomy
	Post-surgical (hernia, scrotal surgery)
	Congenital absence of vas (CABVD)
Ejaculatory duct obstruction	Post-surgical
	Mullerian cysts
	Post-infective

should be recorded as well as whether she has been investigated. The pertinent points in the history allow the clinician to identify whether the underlying cause is primary or secondary infertility and also whether this is non-obstructive or obstructive. In this particular case the male has never fathered a child and therefore presents with primary infertility. The other relevant points are the previous orchidopexy and the presence of a varicocoele.

In obstructive cases the underlying obstruction can occur anywhere from the efferent tubules to the ejaculatory ducts. The obstruction may be congenital, such as Mullerian duct cysts or Wolffian duct abnormalities, causing ejaculatory duct obstruction or congenital bilateral absence of vas (CBAVD). Acquired causes include sexually transmitted infections causing strictures within the epididymi and vas or surgical trauma. The common causes of obstructive azoospermia are listed in Table 3.1.

The sexual history should record any previous pregnancies or miscarriages and also include the frequency and timing of intercourse with the female cycle. Any history of erectile dysfunction or premature ejaculation should also be recorded. Previous sexually transmitted infections may result in obstructive azoospermia and an STD screen should be performed to ensure that there is no underlying active chlamydia infection. Excessive alcohol, smoking and illicit drug use, are factors which may reduce the sperm count in male patients. Male patients undergoing chemotherapy or treatment with gonadotoxic agents can develop azoospermia which may persist for several years following treatment before recovering. In cases of non-obstructive azoospermia, surgical reconstruction is not feasible. Common causes of non-obstructive azoospermia are listed in Table 3.2.

Table 3.2 Causes of non-obstructive azoospermia.

Germinal aplasia	Radiotherapy
	Chemotherapy
	Drug-induced
	Klinefelter's syndrome
	XYY syndrome
	Idiopathic
Maturation arrest	Idiopathic
	XYY syndrome
	Varicocoele
Endocrine abnormalities	Pituitary disease
	Hypogonadotrophic hypogonadism
	Hyperprolactinaemia
	Oestrogens
Genetic abnormalities	Kallman's syndrome
	XX male
	Androgen insensitivity syndrome
	5-alpha reductase deficiency
	Noonan's syndrome
	Down's syndrome
	XYY syndrome

Examination

A general examination to evaluate the general stature and secondary sexual characteristics is conducted to ensure that the endocrine status of the patient is normal. The inguinal areas are checked for scars which may indicate previous hernia repairs or orchidopexy for cryptorchidism. The testicular volume should be greater than 15 ml and small testicles are a sign of testicular failure. The presence of dilated epididymi may indicate obstruction or can be secondary to previous infection. The vasa are palpated bilaterally to ensure that they are present. In obstructive azoospermia, a rectal examination is performed to define and evaluate the prostate gland which should be of a smooth consistency. The patient is then examined standing up in order to detect the presence of a varicocoele.

Table 3.3 WHO criteria for normal semen analysis.

Volume	≥ 2 ml
pH	7.0–8.0
Sperm concentration	20 million/ml
Motility	>50% forward progressive motility
Morphology	≥ 14% normal shape and form
Leucocytes	< 1 million/ml

Investigations

Investigations are guided by the examination and the semen analysis. The semen analysis is conducted following at least two days of abstinence (otherwise semen volume is reduced), but ideally no more than 5 days (as this decreases sperm motility). A standardised counter is used and the results are compared to a WHO reference range shown in Table 3.3.

Oligozoospermia refers to a sperm concentration of less than 20 million/ml. Asthenozoospermia indicates that < 50% of the spermatozoa are motile and teratozoospermia refers to less than 14% normal forms. Quite often all three parameters are abnormal in the same specimen and this is referred to as OATS (oligoazothenoteratospermia) syndrome.

A hormone profile is checked which includes measurement of the serum FSH, LH and testosterone levels. Generally, if the FSH is twice the normal value in the presence of small testicles and azoospermia then the diagnosis is likely to be testicular failure. Elevated FSH, LH levels with low testosterone may indicate primary testicular failure or hypergonadotrophic hypogonadism. A low FSH, LH and testosterone indicates hypogonadotrophic hypogonadism (e.g. Kallman's syndrome) and requires further assessment by an endocrinologist and the offering of hCG therapy.

Investigation of azoospermia

The presence of azoospermia means that the patient has no sperm in the ejaculated sample and will require some form of intervention in order to conceive. It is important to distinguish between obstructive and non-obstructive azoospermia. In a specialised unit a karyotype is performed. Approximately 14% of men with azoospermia and 5% of men with oligozoospermia will have an abnormal karyotype. Therefore patients must be counselled prior to undergoing these tests. Mutations involving the cystic fibrosis transmembrane conductance regulator (CFTR) which is located on chromosome 7 is associated with congenital bilateral absence of vas (CBAVD). Congenital bilateral absence of vas can be detected by palpation and should always be considered in men found to be azoospermic.

Hormone assays, as mentioned above, can give an indication as to whether the underlying cause is obstructive or non-obstructive.

Azoospermia with a low volume ejaculate and a reduced pH may indicate ejaculatory duct obstruction and therefore further investigations in the form of a transrectal ultrasound scan of the prostate (usually arranged after referral to a urologist) can be requested and performed in order to identify the site of the obstruction and the presence of a Mullerian duct cyst.

Management of azoospermia and further discussion

If the underlying aetiology is obstruction, then patients need to be referred to secondary care and can be offered the option of potential reconstructive surgery combined with sperm extraction and storage for later use with assisted techniques if required. The anatomy and patency can be visualised using an injection of contrast directly into the vas and detecting the site of the obstruction and ensuring distal patency. Reconstruction involves a variety of techniques, including vasovasostomy, where the two ends of the vas are anastomosed together, or epididymovasostomy, where the vas is anastomosed directly to a seminiferous tubule. Intra-testicular obstruction is seen in 15% of cases of obstructive azoospermia and is not amenable to reconstruction.

Ejaculatory duct obstruction is managed using a combined approach. A transrectal ultrasound is performed intraoperatively to inject methylene blue dye into the ejaculatory ducts and seminal vesicles. A resectoscope can be used to de-roof a Mullerian duct cyst or blocked ejaculatory ducts until the methylene blue dye flows through the ducts.

If the vasogram shows no obstruction then the diagnosis is impaired spermatogenesis. This is commonly due to two reasons: firstly maturation arrest, in which the spermatocyte development is impaired at certain stages; and secondly Sertoli cell only syndrome. Here the testicle is composed of Sertoli cells, which act as support cells for the developing spermatocytes, but there are no mature sperm. Although these conditions present as azoospermia, microdissection techniques have been successful in retrieving sperm from a proportion of these patients.

Semen analysis may also indicate oligospermia. In this group of patients conservative measures to improve semen parameters are advised, e.g. stop smoking and limit the exposure to gonadotoxins. If a varicocoele is present then an ultrasound is performed to measure the testicular size and confirm the presence of the varicocoele. The management of a varicocoele in the infertile patient is controversial. There are several methods available to correct a varicocoele, including microsurgical inguinal ligation, laparoscopic ligation or radiological embolisation. *Although the semen parameters may improve, this does not necessarily result in a higher paternity rate following correction of the varicocoele.*

Generally, if sperm are present on the semen analysis then intrauterine insemination, *in vitro* fertilisation (IVF) or intracytoplasmic sperm injection (ICSI) can be used as assisted techniques. The treatment of male infertility has greatly advanced since the introduction of ICSI, as this technique utilises micromanipulation techniques to inject a *single* sperm into a mature oocyte. The oocytes are then checked the next day to ensure that fertilisation has occurred. This technique allows assisted reproduction despite very low sperm counts or poor motility.

Sperm retrieval techniques

A variety of techniques are available in order to retrieve sperm for later use in IVF or ICSI. When exploratory surgery is carried out on the azoospermic patient, this is combined with a TESE (testicular exploration and sperm extraction). The tissue obtained is centrifuged in a special medium and sperm harvested and stored for later use. Alternative methods to obtain sperm directly from the testicle include the use of needle aspiration or biopsy needles.

PESA (percutaneous epididymal sperm aspiration) allows direct aspiration of sperm from the epididymis in cases of congenital absence of vas or post-vasectomy patients who do not want to undergo a reversal. As the epididymis is already dilated sperm can be aspirated directly into the medium using a large gauge needle.

MESA (micro-epididymal sperm aspiration) involves an open technique whereby an incision is made into the tubules within the epididymis and sperm are retrieved using an operating microscope.

Although the vas deferens patency rates for patients undergoing a vasectomy reversal approach 90% (note, however, that pregnancy rates are lower), the success rates for epididymovasostomy are much lower, and therefore a large proportion of patients will require some form of assisted conception provided that sperm has been retrieved by the techniques described above. In those patients where sperm retrieval has not been possible the options include the use of donor sperm or adoption.

Review of case history

This particular case involves an azoospermic male with two risk factors: a history of cryptorchidism corrected surgically and the presence of a varicocoele on the opposite side. The orchidopexy as a child could have resulted in a vas deferens injury or stricturing of the vas deferens. This was investigated using a vasogram which showed that the vas was patent throughout its entire length bilaterally. Although the presence of a varicocoele may have an effect on semen parameters, it is unlikely to cause azoospermia. Therefore in this case correction of the varicocoele is not entirely indicated unless the patient is symptomatic or the testicular volume is getting progressively smaller. This patient elected not to have surgery for the varicocoele. Bilateral biopsies of the testicles were performed and a microdissection TESE was used to retrieve sperm. The biopsies suggested Sertoli cell only syndrome, but sperm were successfully retrieved using the microdissection technique. The couple then underwent successful IVF treatment.

Reasons for referral to secondary care

Male infertility has seen significant developments in reconstructive techniques and sperm extraction. Provided that there is sperm available, either via an ejaculated sample or sperm extraction techniques, successful fertilisation can be achieved using IVF techniques. Male patients with abnormal semen parameters presenting with infertility should be referred to secondary care for further assessment as the identification of reversible causes will allow natural conception.

Key points

- Both partners should be investigated when presenting with infertility.
- Male infertility is common and should be initially investigated by means of a semen analysis, endocrine tests and a clinical examination.
- Provided that sperm are present in the ejaculate, assisted reproduction techniques (ICSI and IVF) can be used to achieve successful pregnancies.
- Surgical reconstructive techniques can be used in obstructive azoospermia.
- The use of ICSI has revolutionised the treatment of male factor infertility.

Further reading and bibliography

Lipshultz, L. I., Thomas, A. J. and Khera, M. (2007). Surgical management of male infertility. In: *Campbell-Walsh Urology*, 9th edn (eds. A. J. Wein, L. R. Kavoussi, A. C. Novick, A. W. Partin and C. A. Peters), pp. 654–716. Saunders Elsevier, Philadelphia, PA.

Sigman, M. and Jarow, J. P. (2007) Male infertility. In: *Campbell-Walsh Urology*, 9th edn (eds. A. J. Wein, L. R. Kavoussi, A. C. Novick, A. W. Partin and C. A. Peters), pp. 609–50. Saunders Elsevier, Philadelphia, PA.

CHAPTER 4

Urinary tract infection in adults

Paul Erotocritou, Sima Patel, Neehar Arya, Rizwan Hamid and Petros Erotocritou

Case history

A 33-year-old female presents with complaints of increased urinary frequency and burning pain when urinating. She had suffered from the same symptoms three months earlier, when an *Escherchia coli* urinary infection had been confirmed and which had resolved after a short course of antibiotics.

Introduction

Incidence and epidemiology

A urinary tract infection (UTI) is one of the most frequent presentations to a General Practitioner: 2–3% of all consultations, and even 6% in the case of women, are due to symptoms suggesting UTI.

Apart from neonates, UTIs are more common in females than males. One per cent of schoolgirls have bacteriuria. This increases to 4% in young adults. Around 30% of women aged between 20 and 40 years will have a symptomatic UTI in their lifetime. The ratio of women to men with bacteriuria progressively decreases with age. Once a patient has an infection she is more likely to develop subsequent infections. The probability of recurrent UTIs increases with the number of previous infections. Interestingly, this decreases in inverse proportion to the elapsed time between the two infections

Urinary tract infections – definitions

A UTI can be defined in a variety of ways. Classically, an inflammatory response of the urothelium to bacterial invasion is described as a urinary tract infection. This is usually associated with bacteriuria and pyuria.

Initially it was thought a pure growth bacterial count of $>10^5$ bacteria/ml (or colony forming units/ml) of urine is required to diagnose a UTI. However, now it is agreed that in a symptomatic female a count of 10^2 bacteria/ml pure growth is sufficient for diagnosis.

The various definitions associated with UTI are stated below. UTIs themselves can be classified in three ways:

1. Classification by symptoms:
   - **Cystitis** is a constellation of symptoms consisting of dysuria, frequency, urgency, and suprapubic pain. These symptoms may also be associated with infection of the urethra or vagina or non-infectious conditions such as interstitial cystitis, bladder carcinoma or calculi.
   - **Acute pyelonephritis** is defined as a combination of chills, fever, and flank pain associated with bacteriuria and pyuria.
2. Classification in terms of the anatomic or functional status of the urinary tract and the health of the host:
   - **Uncomplicated UTI**: an infection in a healthy patient with a structurally and functionally normal urinary tract. Women comprise a majority of these patients.
   - **Complicated UTI**: this infection is accompanied by factors that increase the chance of acquiring bacteria and decrease the efficacy of therapy. The urinary tract can be functionally or structurally abnormal. Some of these factors are listed below:
     - Male gender
     - Pregnancy
     - Elderly
     - Diabetes
     - Immunosuppression
     - Indwelling urinary catheter
     - Spinal cord injury
3. Classification by their relationship to other UTIs:
   - **Isolated UTI**: first infection or an infection after an interval of at least six months.
   - **Unresolved UTI**: an infection that has not responded to antimicrobial therapy.
   - **Recurrent UTI**: more than two infections in six months or three in 12 months. This is called **reinfection** when the UTI is caused by different

bacteria. It is known as **bacterial persistence or relapsed UTI** if the infection is by the same organism. Relapsed infection should raise the suspicion of a focus of persistent infection, e.g. urinary tract stones or rarer causes such as urethral diverticulum in a female.

Other important definitions to note are:

- **Bacteriuria** is the presence of bacteria in the urine.
- **Pyuria**, the presence of white blood cells (WBCs) in the urine, is generally indicative of infection and an inflammatory response of the urothelium to the bacterium. Bacteriuria without pyuria is generally indicative of bacterial colonisation without infection of the urinary tract. Pyuria without bacteriuria (sterile pyuria) warrants evaluation for tuberculosis, stones, or cancer or may be the result of a partially treated UTI.
- **Prophylactic antibiotic therapy** is the suppression of a focus of bacterial persistence that cannot be eradicated. A low nightly dosage of an antimicrobial agent usually results in the urine showing no growth.

These definitions require careful clinical and bacteriologic assessment and are important because they influence the type and extent of the patient's evaluation and treatment.

Urinary tract infections – microbiology

Most UTIs are due to faecally derived bacteria. These are facultative anaerobes. The commonest is *Escherichia coli* (*E. coli*), which accounts for 70–85% of community acquired UTIs. Other organisms causing uncomplicated cystitis in the community include *Staphylococcus saprophyticus* (10%), *Enterococcus faecalis* (8%), *Proteus mirabilis* (6%) and *Klebisella* (3%). However, in complicated UTIs *E. coli* only accounts for 50% of cases. The remainder are caused by other organisms described above, but also include *Pseudomonas aeruginosa*.

Urinary tract infections – routes

- *Ascending route*: the most common route of UTI is ascending infection. Hence the increased risk in females due to a short urethra. The organisms ascend along the urethra to the bladder.
- *Haematogenous route*: this is the cause of UTIs with *Staphylococcus aureus*, *Candida albicans* and *Mycobacterium tuberculosis*.

■ *Infection via lymphatics*: UTIs are rarely caused by this route. This is usually due to inflammatory bowel disease.

History and examination

A patient with UTI may present with one or all of the following symptoms: frequency, dysuria, urgency, incontinence, strangury (slow painful micturition due to irritation causing spasm of the urethra and bladder). It is also relevant in the history to assess for predisposing factors such as sexual activity, contraceptive use and pregnancy.

On examination the patient may have haematuria or foul-smelling urine. Suprapubic or lower abdominal tenderness may be present in cases of cystitis and there may also be vaginal irritation or discharge. Renal angle tenderness with pyrexia would suggest pyelonephritis.

Investigations

Urine collection

Prior to considering urinary investigations one must discuss the method of urine collection, as diagnostic accuracy is greatly affected by the method and the attention to detail in collecting the urine sample. In primary care it is generally feasible to collect only voided specimens rather than those obtained by catheterisation or suprapubic aspiration.

Voided specimens

Women: the female should be instructed to spread the labia and cleanse the peri-urethral area with a moist gauze. Importantly, the gauze should be moved from urethra downwards to avoid contamination. Antiseptics should not be used as they may cause contamination and lead to false-negative culture. The first 10 ml of urine is discarded and a midstream specimen, which is representative of the bladder, is collected.

Men: no preparation is required in circumcised men. In uncircumcised men the foreskin should be retracted and the glans cleaned with soap and rinsed before collection of specimen. A midstream urine specimen should then be collected, as described above.

Catheterised specimens

If the woman has difficulty in spreading and maintaining separation of the labia, then a catheterised specimen should be obtained. A mid-catheterised specimen can be collected.

Suprapubic aspiration

This is the most accurate method of obtaining a urine specimen. However, this carries some morbidity and there is limited clinical usefulness. This method is particularly useful in cases where repeated cultures are negative but the patient has pyuria. A full bladder is ensured and the suprapubic area cleaned with a swab. After instillation of local anaesthesia, a 20 ml syringe is used to aspirate 5 ml for culture and 15 ml of urine for centrifugation and urinalysis.

Urinary investigations

Urine dipstix of midstream urine specimen

This simple test can be used to detect red cells, white cells, leucocyte esterase and nitrites. However, although a simple test, an understanding of the dynamics is necessary.

- Red cells may be detected in the presence of UTI due to inflammation of the urothelium.
- White blood cells in the urine (pyuria), suggests inflammation of the urothelium. This can be due to bacteria; however, there are other causes for pyuria in the absence of bacteria, such as urinary tract stones and carcinoma *in situ* of the urothelium. Leucocyte esterase is produced by neutrophils and consequently detects the presence of white blood cells in the urine. However, not all patients with bacteria in their urine (bacteriuria) have significant pyuria. The sensitivity of this dipstix test for the detection of infection is 70–95%, meaning that 5–30% of patients with an infection will have a dipstix negative for leucocyte esterase.

■ Nitrite testing on dipstix is for indirect detection of bacteria in the urine, utilising the fact that nitrites are not normally found in the urine and that some bacteria can convert nitrates into nitrites. The sensitivity of nitrite dipstix detection is 35–85% whilst the specificity is 92–100%. This means that if the nitrite test is positive the patient is likely to have a UTI, but a negative test often occurs although an infection is present. The combination of the nitrite test with leukocyte esterase with a positive result on either is more specific but less sensitive than either test alone (sensitivity 75–84%, specificity 82–98%).

Consequently it is not necessary for a urine dipstix to test positive for all features to confirm a UTI. For instance, a sample which is positive for white cells and nitrites is very likely to be infected as is a sample which is only positive for nitrites.

Microscopy and culture of midstream urine (MSU) specimen

Microscopy is a useful diagnostic tool in patients with urinary symptoms. White cells can be seen and up to three white cells per high-power field is considered normal. The absence of a significant number of white cells in urine should make one doubt UTI as a diagnosis. Bacteria may also be seen in the urine. However, this technique is not void from being subject to false results. False negatives can occur when there are low bacterial counts, making it difficult to identify bacteria, whilst false positives can occur due to contamination of the sample with commensal bacteria of the distal urethra or perineum and also the ability of bacteria to multiply rapidly in urine standing at room temperature. Bacteria noted on a microscopic examination should be interpreted in view of clinical signs and symptoms of urinary tract infection. Diagnosis of bacteriuria in a patient with a suspected urinary tract infection requires a urine culture and sensitivity.

Urine culture is thought of as the 'gold standard' investigation for the diagnosis of UTI, although problems exist for this technique as it relies on the urine being collected properly and cultured quickly. Traditionally a diagnosis of UTI was based on finding of a pure growth of 10^5 bacteria/ml of urine. However, many women with symptoms of UTI present with much lower bacterial counts (10^2–10^3 bacteria/ml pure growth), whilst patients with asymptomatic bacteriuria can have much higher counts. As a result the requirement of a count of 10^5 bacteria/ml of urine is no longer required to make a diagnosis of UTI, and in a symptomatic patient a pure growth of 10^2–10^3 bacteria/ml is suggestive of UTI. It should be noted that a mixed growth is indicative of contamination.

Other investigations

Further investigations are indicated in those patients with recurrent relapsed (persistent) infections (i.e. multiple infections with the same organism), as this suggests pathology within the urinary tract. For example, an ultrasound scan of the urinary tract combined with a plain X-ray may be requested to exclude stones, and in females a urethral diverticulum may be diagnosed with an MRI scan.

Management and discussion

Uncomplicated UTI

For an episode of isolated uncomplicated UTI, an excellent response can be gained from empirical treatment with trimethoprim or nitrofurantoin. This is generally given for 3–5 days. This treatment is administered before culture sensitivities are available. If symptoms were to persist antibiotic therapy could be changed according to sensitivities (see Table 4.1 for dosing regimes). In cases not responding to the above, ciprofloxacin is usually very effective as the second line.

Recurrent UTI – reinfection

Recurrent UTIs due to reinfection with different organisms (see definitions above) are common in healthy young women, although they have a structurally and functionally normal urinary tract. As already mentioned, UTIs in women are thought to represent ascending infections, with bacteria

Table 4.1 Oral antibiotic agents for treating UTI and UTI prophylaxis.

Agent	Dose/frequency	Use
Trimethoprim	200 mg BD 3–5 days	Active infection
Trimethoprim	100 mg nocte	Prophylaxis
Nitrofurantoin	50 mg/100 mg BD/QDS 3–5 days	Active infection
Nitrofurantoin	50–100 mg nocte	Prophylaxis
Ciprofloxacin	250–500mg BD 3–5 days	Active infection

colonising the perineum and ascending the short female urethra with ease, causing a symptomatic UTI. It is because of this mechanism that sexual intercourse is thought to play a role, with sexual activity causing bacteria from the vagina to be pushed up the urethra into the bladder. However, although intercourse may play a role in women susceptible to UTI, but the fact that most sexually active women do not get UTIs argues against its role as a primary mechanism. Other evidence suggests that young women with recurrent reinfection have a hereditary susceptibility to these infections (increased HLA-A3 prevalence in this group).

These patients should be given general advice regarding the avoidance of scented or bubble baths, regular bladder emptying and adequate fluid intake of at least two litres per day (avoid caffeinated drinks). They may also benefit from cranberry juice, which has been shown to decrease symptomatic recurrences of UTIs by prevention of *E. coli* adherence to the urothelium. Ingestion of bio yogurt increases commensal lactobacilli in the vaginal flora, creating an acidic environment in this area and thus hindering bacterial colonisation of the vagina, which is thought to precede urethral and bladder involvement. In females where infections are related to intercourse, voiding post-intercourse and avoidance of spermicides and tampons can be helpful. Spermicides, whether they be used on a diaphragm or a condom, may enhance *E. coli* adherence to urothelial cells through reducing natural vaginal flora.

In addition to these measures three specific options are available:

1. In patients where it appears recurrence of UTI is related to intercourse, antibiotics can be taken after intercourse (post-coital prophylaxis).
2. Women who suffer from infrequent reinfections (> 4 per year) can be given a course of antibiotics or a prescription to initiate self-medication when symptoms of UTI recur (patient-initiated antibiotic therapy).
3. The final option is low-dose antibiotic prophylaxis for women who suffer more than four UTIs a year, as this will help prevent infection and can lead to the resolution of perineal colonisation with uropathogens. The common antibiotics and regimes are shown in Table 4.1.

Recurrent UTI – relapsed (persistent)

As previously discussed, recurrent relapsed (persistent) infections (i.e. multiple infections with the same organism) suggests pathology within the urinary tract. This group needs focused investigations to elucidate the cause, which is then managed appropriately.

UTI in pregnancy

Urinary infections are not uncommon in pregnancy: 20–40% of females with asymptomatic bacteriuria will develop pyelonephritis during pregnancy. Hence pregnancy is one condition where asymptomatic bacteriuria should be treated. The safe antibiotics during pregnancy are penicillins and cephalosporins. Nitrofurantoin can be used in the first and second trimesters only.

The antibiotics to avoid during pregnancy are:

- Tetracyclines   all trimesters
- Quinolones   all trimesters
- Trimethoprim   first trimester
- Aminoglycosides   second and third trimesters
- Chloramphenicol   third trimester
- Sulphonamide   third trimester
- Nitrofurantoin   third trimester

Once the treatment has been completed a negative culture must be confirmed, unlike in simple uncomplicated UTI, where this is not necessary. In case of recurrent UTIs in pregnancy a low dose of cephalexin, 125–250 mg daily, is effective.

UTI in post-menopausal women

The antibiotics policy is the same as for pre-menopausal women. However, the use of short-term therapy is not well established. Also, in case of recurrent UTIs further urological and gynaecological investigations should be performed to rule out bladder malignancy, obstruction or detrusor failure. Importantly, in this group the use of intravaginal oestrogens has been shown to reduce the rate of recurrent infections considerably, as they help to reverse atrophic vaginal epithelial changes and thus promote colonisation of this region with normal commensals (lactobacilli).

Acute pyelonephritis

This is defined as an infectious inflammation of the renal parenchyma and collecting system. It should be suspected in those patients with fever, rigors, loin pain and lower urinary tract symptoms (dysuria, frequency, urgency). It is important to rule out underlying causes by necessary investigations and initial intravenous antibiotics are essential due to the potential of serious complications (e.g. septic shock, pyelonephrosis and renal abscess). For these reasons these patients should be referred immediately to secondary care.

Key points

■ Urinary tract infection is a common problem which can be dealt with effectively in primary care, when uncomplicated.
■ Complicated and recurrent relapsed (persistent) UTIs when identified should be referred for definitive treatment to a urologist due to the possibility of underlying pathology and significant morbidity.
■ Clinicians can make a diagnosis of UTI confidently from history, examination and urine dipstix.
■ Broad spectrum antibiotic therapy should be initiated according to local recommendations on sensitivities.
■ It is important that, if urine culture shows the need for selective antibiotics to be used, they are initiated.

Further reading and bibliography

European Association of Urology Guidelines (2008) http://www.uroweb.org/professional-resources/guidelines/; accessed June 2008.

Nazareth, I. and King, M. (1993) Decision making by general practitioners in diagnosis and management of lower urinary tract symptoms in women. *Br. Med. J.*, **306**, 1103–6.

Ramakrishnan, K. and Scheid, D. C. (2005) Diagnosis and management of acute pyelonephritis in adults. *Am. Fam. Physician.*, **71**, 933–42.

Semeniuk, H. and Church, D. (1999) Evaluation of the leukocyte esterase and nitrite urine dipstick screening tests for detection of bacteriuria in women with suspected uncomplicated urinary tract infections. *J. Clin. Microbiol.*, **37**, 3051–2.

Sheffield, J. S. and Cunningham, F. G. (2005) Urinary tract infection in women. *Obstet. Gynecol.*, **106**, 1085–92.

CHAPTER 5

Overactive bladder, urgency and stress urinary incontinence in adult females

Pippa Sangster, Miles Goldstraw, Rajesh Kavia, Ketan Kansagra, Vinay Kalsi and Rizwan Hamid

Case history

A 65-year-old woman comes to the GP's surgery for follow-up of hypertension. Her medical history is otherwise unremarkable and current medication includes a beta-blocker. She has three grown children who were all normal vaginal deliveries. She reports she has been having some accidental loss of urine for several years and has recently heard from a friend that there may be treatment options. Both she and her GP decide to evaluate this issue further and schedule an appointment for the following week. Following a detailed history, examination and routine investigations, a diagnosis of overactive bladder syndrome resulting in urgency incontinence was made. She was given advice regarding lifestyle changes and bladder retraining, and commenced on Solifenacin 5 mg OD. Her symptoms improved significantly.

Introduction

Urinary incontinence (UI) is defined by the International Continence Society as 'a complaint of any involuntary loss of urine'. Suffering from UI is not only distressing, but it has a negative impact on patients' quality of life through a loss of dignity and imposed limitations on lifestyles. Due to the perceived anti-social and embarrassing nature of this complaint it is rather under-reported. However, it is a common condition, with a suggested prevalence of more than one in three adults over the age of 40 having clinically significant symptoms of this nature. This has considerable financial implications and The Continence Foundation has estimated a total cost for the United Kingdom (UK) of more than £420 million (approximately 1/120th of the total expenditure of the NHS).

UI can affect both sexes. In males, it is mainly secondary to benign prostatic hyperplasia or occurs following major prostatic surgery. Male incontinence will not be further discussed in this chapter.

Classification

It is important at the outset to define the various terms related to urinary incontinence accurately. This not only helps to diagnose a particular condition but also leads to effective and appropriate treatment and improves communication between the various health care providers.

- **Overactive bladder syndrome**: a syndrome characterised by urgency with or without incontinence, usually accompanied with frequency and nocturia. The underlying pathology of this condition is presumed to be **idiopathic detrusor overactivity/instability**.
- **Urgency**: a sudden compelling desire to pass urine that cannot be deferred.
- **Urge incontinence**: involuntary leakage of urine accompanied by or immediately preceded by urgency. Usually represents a severe form of overactive bladder syndrome.
- **Stress urinary incontinence**: involuntary leakage of urine on effort or exertion, or on coughing or sneezing.
- **Mixed urinary incontinence**: involuntary leakage of urine associated with urgency and also with exertion, effort, sneezing and coughing.

Although UI is a concern for individuals of all ages, stress UI is the prominent type of incontinence among younger women (< 65 years) and as women age urgency UI becomes more prevalent. This older age group (≥ 65 years) make up approximately two-thirds to three-quarters of reported cases of incontinence.

Table 5.1 Causes of transient urinary incontinence.

Drugs (e.g. sedatives)
Constipation with impacted faeces
Acute confusional state
Restricted mobility
Urinary tract infection
Atrophic vaginitis
Increased urine output (e.g. heart failure, diuretics, hyperglycaemia)
Psychological dysfunction

Assessment

When assessing patients for UI there are certain key questions that need to be considered:

- Is incontinence long-standing or transient? Transient UI may be related to a treatable isolated event, the causes of which are listed in Table 5.1.
- Is there any underlying medical condition that may be causing the incontinence?
- Is there any voiding dysfunction causing overflow incontinence?
- Is this stress or urgency incontinence, and if there are mixed symptoms, which is the most distressing symptom?
- Are there any special problems which will need referral to a urologist or uro-gynaecologist?

History

A focused history of the complaint should include the nature and impact of incontinence symptoms. Lower urinary tract symptoms (LUTS) which may accompany UI, together with possible underlying causes, are detailed in Table 5.2. On direct questioning it is possible to gauge the nature of UI; urine leakage with exertion, coughing or sneezing is generally due to stress incontinence whilst incontinence with urinary frequency, urgency and nocturia points towards urgency incontinence. The volume of urine loss can also provide valuable information as to the nature of incontinence; urgency incontinence is more likely to be associated with a large loss

Table 5.2 Definitions of several lower urinary tract symptoms (LUTS) and their possible causes.

Lower urinary tract symptom	Definition (*National Institute of Health*)	Causes
Increased daytime frequency	Complaint of voiding too often during the day (*voids more than 8 times/24 hours*)	■ Excessive fluid intake ■ Overactive bladder syndrome/ detrusor overactivity due to a relevant neurological condition or where there is no defined cause (idiopathic)
Nocturia	Complaint that the individual has to wake up one or more times to void (*the patient wakes from sleep to pass urine*)	■ Impaired bladder compliance ■ Bladder outlet obstruction due to prostatic problems; uro-genital prolapse; urethral stricture; following bladder neck surgery
Urgency	Complaint of a sudden compelling desire to void which is difficult to defer (*patient feels a strong need to pass urine for fear of leakage*)	■ Increased bladder sensation ■ Urinary tract infection ■ Bladder tumour ■ Renal tract stones ■ Interstitial cystitis

of urine, whereas the amount lost with stress incontinence tends to be small. The history should also include a gynaecological and obstetric history, relevant coexisting medical conditions (e.g. diabetes, hypertension, multiple sclerosis, stroke, dementia, Parkinsonism and arthritis), current medication and a functional status including any sensory or mobility problems. History of any other pelvic organ dysfunction, such as bowel or sexual dysfunction, may be relevant, as these could be associated with or contributing to UI. A review of environmental factors (social, cultural and physical) and lifestyle factors (exercise and fluid intake), previous treatment history together with current goals and expectations is also important.

Quality of life disease-specific questionnaires ,such as the King's Health questionnaire, are useful in determining the impact of bladder symptoms on quality of life, and subsequent questionnaires may be used to assess the success of any intervention. These questionnaires, however, are often provided only in secondary care, but may be used by GPs who have a specialist interest in this condition.

Examination

Physical examination is an essential component of the assessment because it can detect modifiable factors or associated conditions and help determine the type of UI. The general examination should include abdominal and gynaecological examinations and in specific cases where there may be a neurological cause a neurological assessment, including rectal/anal examination, is performed. The abdominal examination will reveal scars from previous surgery as well as the presence of organomegaly or a palpable bladder. The gynaecological examination includes examination of the external genitalia, vagina and the perineum to look for excoriations, masses, prolapse and abnormal perineal sensation. The pelvic floor muscle strength can also be assessed while the examiner is performing a digital vaginal examination. A stress test can be performed by asking the patient to cough whilst examining the urethral meatus. The neurological examination should focus on an assessment of gait, abduction and dorsiflexion of the toes (S3), sensation of the sole and lateral aspect of the thigh (S2) and the perineum (S3). A rectal examination will provide a subjective assessment of resting and voluntary anal tone (S2–S4).

Investigations

In order to complete the assessment there are certain straightforward investigations that can be performed in the surgery which will enable the GP to make an accurate diagnosis and start the most appropriate treatment.

Dipstix urinalysis

This is a quick, easy and cheap test that can be carried out which could sometimes eliminate the need for more expensive investigations. Reagent strips demonstrate the presence of haemoglobin, leucocyte esterase (present in pyuria), nitrites (present in bacterial infection), protein (present with glomerular disease or infection) and glucose (present in poorly controlled or undiagnosed diabetes).

Midstream urine (MSU)

In the face of a positive urinalysis an MSU should be sent for microscopy, culture and sensitivities. Symptomatic patients with a proven UTI may then be treated with the appropriate antibiotic according to the sensitivities.

Urine cytology

Urine may be sent for cytology to look for any atypical cells (bladder tumour may result in urgency and urge incontinence). This should be routinely done if there is any haematuria present, either gross or on dipstix. Without haematuria the diagnostic value of cytology is generally poor.

Bladder diary

A bladder diary or a frequency–volume chart is an extremely useful tool in objectively assessing a patient's urinary complaint as well as the degree of UI and the circumstances associated with it. The diurnal variation in voided volumes can also be assessed. The patient records the time and volume of each urinary void and any incontinence episodes experienced. Studies have shown that a bladder diary kept over three days provides the most useful information to the clinician. By keeping sequential diaries the response to any treatment or intervention can also be monitored.

Pad testing

This test is usually requested by a urologist or a GP with a specialist interest. It is performed by a specialist nurse and used if there is doubt about the existence or degree of incontinence. Continence pads are continually worn for a set period of time and subsequently weighed on their removal for any abnormal increase (>8 grams/24 hours) in pad weight.

Referral to urology/uro-gynaecology

If after completing an initial assessment the type of UI remains unclear, a referral to a urologist or uro-gynaecologist can be considered. The conditions for which other investigations are indicated and a specialist referral necessary are shown in Table 5.3.

Table 5.3 Indications for specialist referral.

1. Recurrent urinary tract infections
2. Haematuria
3. Evidence of impaired renal function
4. Pain thought to be arising from the upper or lower urinary tract
5. Significant post-micturition residual volume
6. Significant pelvic organ prolapse
7. History of pelvic irradiation
8. History of radical pelvic surgery
9. Suspected fistula
10. Suspected neurological cause of incontinence
11. Failure of initial treatment

Management and discussion

It has already been established that stress and urgency incontinence are completely separate entities and as such their treatment options will differ. With mixed incontinence the management is dictated by which form of incontinence is the dominant one and this one should be treated first. It is important to counsel these patients that the lesser form of incontinence may remain and be troublesome. Management of all forms of incontinence should start off with conservative methods followed by more invasive treatment options if necessary. It should be noted that the management of urgency incontinence and overactive bladder is very similar, as urgency incontinence is usually due to a severe form of overactive bladder syndrome.

Management common to both stress and urge incontinence

For both stress and urgency incontinence there are certain preventative lifestyle changes that can be recommended. Obesity is an independent risk factor for UI and there is a body of evidence to suggest that weight loss in obese women decreases incontinence. A reduction in smoking, caffeine and alcohol intake, and a moderation in fluid intake may improve continence. Ensuring a balanced diet and avoiding constipation is beneficial, as chronic straining when at stool may be a risk factor for pelvic organ prolapse and UI.

Management of stress incontinence

Physiotherapy

The continence mechanism can be reinforced by identifying and exercising the pelvic floor musculature (Kegel's exercises). This requires a motivated patient and good supervision. This should be tried for a minimum of three months.

Biofeedback

This process provides patients with increased sensory awareness of the pelvic floor musculature through electromyography or pressure measurements. The patient is then able to learn how to better contract and relax the pelvic muscles, thereby improving urinary control. This should be tried for a period of six weeks.

Oral pharmacotherapy

Hormone replacement therapy in post-menopausal women will increase the integrity of tissues supporting the pelvic organs and the vagina; however, there is no evidence that oestrogens alone are useful for the management of incontinence. Duloxetine is a combined norepinephrine and serotonin reuptake inhibitor which in animal models has been shown to significantly increase sphincter muscle activity in the storage phase of the micturition cycle. However, this is not recommended as a first line treatment for stress UI. It is also not recommended as a routine second line treatment.

Surgery

Patients will require specialist referral if they are to be considered for any surgical management for stress incontinence, whether it is for the repair of pelvic organ prolapse or support of the bladder neck. Any patient undergoing invasive surgery for stress incontinence will require assessment with urodynamics preoperatively and counselling regarding outcomes and potential complications such as voiding dysfunction. It is not in the remit of this chapter to look at surgical options in detail, but an indication of the range of interventions is provided below.

1. Burch colposuspension: retropubic elevation and stabilisation of urethra and bladder neck by elevation of vagina.
2. Tension-free vaginal tape (TVT): tape is used to elevate and reposition the urethra and to a certain extent compress the urethra to increase resistance to bladder outlet.
3. Transobturator tape (TOT): an alternative to the TVT. The TOT is introduced via a needle through the obturator foramen.
4. Periurethral bulking agents: these are placed intramurally on either side of the urethra. These are expensive and can achieve continence rates of 30–50% only.
5. Artificial urethral sphincter: considered when other treatment options have failed. These artificial sphincters are expensive and have a high complication rate, requiring frequent revisions.
6. Procedures for associated prolapse:
   - Anterior colporrhaphy: to correct anterior vaginal wall prolapse (cystocele).
   - Posterior colporrhaphy: to correct posterior vaginal wall prolapse (rectocele).
   - Manchester repair: amputation of cervix together with an anterior repair.
   - Sacrospinous fixation: to correct vaginal vault prolapse vaginally.
   - Sacrocolpopexy: to correct vaginal vault prolapse abdominally.

Management of overactive bladder and urge incontinence

Lifestyle changes

The patient is advised to avoid caffeinated beverages and fizzy drinks. They should also avoid alcohol and smoking. Some patient can benefit by avoidance of foods with chillies.

Bladder training

This behavioural technique alters drinking patterns in order to consume less before travelling or going to bed whilst 're-training' to hold on and reduce the symptoms of urgency and frequency. This is tried for a minimum period of six weeks.

Oral pharmacotherapy

Anti-cholinergic agents are a logical first treatment choice in patients with symptoms of overactive bladder. They are generally effective in about 60–80% of patients. The common side-effects of muscarinic receptor blockade include a dry mouth, heartburn, constipation, blurred vision and drowsiness. They are contraindicated in those patients with acute angle glaucoma. According to NICE guidelines, generic oxybutynin should be tried as a first line. However, in clinical experience a significant number of patients do not tolerate the side effects of the medication well. Generally the more selective agents are much better tolerated. Solifenacin and tolterodine are the main anti-cholinergic agents in clinical use at present. In a large clinical trial when these two drugs were directly compared (STAR trial), Solifenacin, with a flexible dosing regimen, showed greater efficacy as compared to tolterodine in decreasing urgency episodes, incontinence, urge incontinence and pad usage and increasing the volume voided per micturition. The side effects were low and comparable in both drugs. Hence, now more and more hospitals have now adopted Solifenacin as their first line anti-cholinergic based on its efficacy.

Table 5.4 lists various agents now available to treat symptoms of detrusor over activity. The long-acting (extended life 'XL') formulation of these medications can be an advantage for patients as they need only take the tablet once a day to provide 24 hour cover for symptoms.

There are theoretical concerns that these medicines may increase the post-void residual urine volume and precipitate acute urinary retention, although in clinical practice this is rarely seen. However, the patients should be evaluated for this problem if after initiation of anti-cholinergics the patient reports slowing of the urinary stream or develops recurrent urinary tract infections.

Surgery

As with stress incontinence patients who have failed first line management must be referred for specialist care. Complex investigations into bladder function/voiding dysfunction such as urodynamics or videourodynamics should be performed in these patients. These investigations will help elucidation of the underlying pathophysiology of the bladder complaint and also provide a baseline in order to gauge the efficacy of the intervention.

1. Detrusor injections of Botulinum Toxin type A: the discovery that injection of Botulinum Toxin A directly into the smooth muscle of the detrusor by a Swiss group resulted in a significant improvement in neurogenic bladder

Table 5.4 Drugs used in overactive bladder.

Generic name	Trade name	Dose (mg)	Frequency	Receptor subtype selectivity	Active metabolite	Elimination half-life of drug (hours)
Propantheline	Pro-Banthine	15	tds	Non-selective	No	<2
Tolterodine tartrate	Detrusitol	2	bd	Non-selective	Yes	2.4
Tolterodine tartrate	Detrusitol XL	4	od	Non-selective	Yes	8.4
Trospium chloride	Regurin	20	bd	Non-selective	No	20
Oxybutynin chloride	Ditropan	2.5–5	bd–qds	Non-selective	Yes	2.3
Oxybutynin chloride XL	Lyrinel XL	5–30	od	Non-selective	Yes	13.2
Propiverine hydrochloride	Detrunorm	15	od–qds	Non-selective	Yes	4.1
Darifenacin	Emselex	7.5–15	od	Selective muscarinic M3 receptor antagonist	Yes	3.1
Solifenacin	Vesicare	5–10	od	Selective muscarinic M2 and M3 receptor antagonist	Yes	40–68

Key: od – once daily; bd – twice daily; tds – three times daily; qds – four times daily; XL – extended life dysfunction is having far reaching consequences in the management of overactive bladder and urgency incontinence. The rational of the treatment was on the basis that Botulinum Toxin A would block the pre-synaptic release of parasympathetic acetylcholine mediating detrusor contraction. The benefits of this treatment appear to exceed those expected from an agent which merely paralyses the detrusor. It seems likely that Botulinum Toxin A is also affecting the vesicular release of neurotransmitters involved in the afferent arm of reflex bladder contractions.

The toxin can be injected under local anaesthesia using a minimally invasive technique with a flexible cystoscope, a procedure which is safe and well tolerated. Patients must be made aware of the fact that there is a risk that they may need to aid bladder emptying by performing clean intermittent self catheterisation (CISC) post treatment. The beneficial effects of the treatment last an average of 10 months. Results of repeated injections demonstrate similar beneficial effects and duration of action of the treatment being comparable to the first injections. Although as yet unlicensed, Botulinum Toxin A is now emerging as the preferred second line treatment (i.e. if anti-cholinergic medication fails) of symptoms of the overactive bladder, and is increasingly being adopted by many urology, neurology and rehabilitation centres worldwide.

2. Sacral neuromodulation: this procedure is only carried out in very specialist centres and involves placing a stimulator implant at the S3 nerve root via its corresponding foramen. Its exact mechanism of action is not fully understood, but it is believed to act on afferent nerve fibres of the bladder which modulate detrusor reflexes and suppress bladder contractions. Neuromodulation is expensive and requires intensive follow-up and patient involvement.

3. 'Clam' cystoplasty: this is a type of augmentation cystoplasty that involves bivalving the bladder to the trigone like a clam and interposing a segment of ileum or colon on its vascular pedicle. It interrupts nervous conduction through detrusor muscle and thus decreases overactive or unstable contractions. This procedure is not without its complications and 60% of patients will need to perform intermittent self-catheterisation post-operatively. Until the advent of minimally invasive treatment options, such as detrusor injections of Botulinum Toxin, this was the mainstay of surgical management of urgency incontinence as a consequence of detrusor overactivity (instability).

4. Urinary diversion: these procedures involve re-diverting urinary drainage from the bladder to either a stoma or a catheterisable continent pouch. Urinary diversion procedures are a last resort for intractable incontinence, but are seldom necessary.

Conclusion

Urinary incontinence of whatever aetiology is likely to have a very negative impact on patients' quality of life. However, much can now be done to improve bladder control. Correct assessment through fastidious history taking and physical examination is generally straightforward and its importance cannot be overemphasised. The development of more selective oral agents is to be welcomed, as is the exciting discovery of intradetrusor Botulinum Neurotoxin A injections to treat severely affected cases of urgency incontinence where there was a paucity of effective second line treatments. Many patients' bladder problems are now being managed initially in a primary care setting, although specialist invention may still be necessary if conservative measures fail. Overall, the options for management of UI have improved greatly in recent years and more patients are able to receive effective treatment for very distressing symptoms.

Key points

- Urinary incontinence is extremely prevalent and represents a huge drain on health resources.
- Many patients never seek medical advice.
- Be aware that there may be an underlying medical cause that could be responsible for UI.
- Judicial and prompt referral to urology/uro-gynaecology is needed as dictated by the patient's history or response to initial treatment.

Further reading and bibliography

Chapple, C. R., Martinez-Garcia, R., Selvaggi, L., Toozs-Hobson, P., Warnack, W., Drogendijk, T., Wright, D. M. and Bolodeoku, J. for the STAR study group (2005) A comparison of the efficacy and tolerability of solifenacin succinate and extended release tolterodine at treating overactive bladder syndrome: results of the STAR trial. *Eur. Urol.*, **48**, 464–70.

European Association of Urology Guidelines, 2008 edition. http://www.uroweb.org/professional-resources/guidelines/; accessed June 2008.

CHAPTER 6

Benign conditions of the scrotum and testis

Davendra Sharma, Gus Cabre and Philippe Grange

Case history

A 28-year-old male patient presents with a painless right testicular lump. He is otherwise well with no significant medical history. Further questioning reveals that the swelling has been present for at least two years but has recently become 'uncomfortable'. How would you assess this gentleman and what is the differential diagnosis?

Introduction

Most 'lumps in the testicle' are in fact benign scrotal conditions, a common reason for patients to consult their GP. Recent campaigns to promote self-examination for testicular cancer have increased this likelihood. The commonest conditions seen include hydrocoeles, epididymal cysts, varicocoeles and skin lesions of the scrotum. We will outline the basic diagnostic principles of scrotal lumps and then discuss the individual conditions. Testicular torsion, a surgical emergency, will be dealt with at the end of this chapter.

Anatomy

The scrotum and testes are part of the male external genitalia. The scrotum is an out pouching of skin and fascia from the perineum. The testes are contained within the scrotum at a temperature which is a few degrees lower than normal body temperature. They consist primarily of seminiferous tubules, where sperm growth and maturation takes place. Adjacent to these tubules are Leydig cells, which produce testosterone.

The epididymis, situated above and behind the testis, is in continuity with the seminiferous tubules and acts as a store and transit for more mature sperm. Sperm travel upwards via the vas deferens towards the ejaculatory duct located in the prostate. The vas deferens is located within the spermatic cord, which also contains the blood supply, nerves and lymphatic drainage of each testis. During development, the testis descends from the abdomen, taking with it several fascial and membranous layers. The most important of these is the tunica vaginalis, which is the obliterated remnant of the processus vaginalis, and which partially surrounds the testis.

Generic approach to the management of scrotal conditions

History

A routine history should include time of onset, duration, change in size or colour, pain, associated trauma or infection, associated lumps, previous episodes and any urological history. Risk factors for testicular cancer such as undescended testes, previous surgery and a positive family history should be included.

Examination

A specific examination to assess the lump – site, size, texture, tenderness, colour, and associated lumps – as well as a general examination is essential. The ability to get above the lump excludes an inguinal origin. Trans-illumination suggests fluid content.

In the case of testicular lumps, the most important examination finding is site. Lumps that are *not* located within the body of the testis are invariably benign. These make up the vast majority of scrotal lumps and will be covered in this chapter (Table 6.1). Lumps located in the body of the testis should be suspected as being malignant and should be referred urgently.

Table 6.1 The differential diagnosis of scrotal pathology.

Structure	Differential diagnosis			
Skin	Lipoma or sebaceous cyst			
	Idiopathic scrotal oedema, Henoch–Schönlein purpura			
Testis or epididymis	Painful	Testicular torsion		
		Epididymo-orchitis		
	Not painful	Cannot get above lump	Hernia	
		Can get above lump	Testis not separate	Testicular tumour
			Testis separate	Epididymal cyst
				Varicocoele
				Hydrocoele

Investigations

The correct diagnosis of most scrotal lumps can be made from the clinical assessment. If there is any doubt or concern, then an ultrasound scan offers excellent definition of the intra-scrotal structures.

Management and discussion (specific to each condition)

Idiopathic hydrocoele

Ninety per cent of hydrocoeles are idiopathic and 10% are secondary to some other pathology. This section refers only to idiopathic hydrocoeles. A hydrocoele is due to the collection of fluid within the tunica vaginalis lining of the testis. The exact aetiology is unclear. In the adult male it is probably due to a change in lymph dynamics – either obstruction of lymphatic channels or overproduction of lymph locally, or a combination of both factors. In tropical countries, 80% of cases are due to filarial infection. In the child it is due to a patent processus vaginalis.

Clinical features

Usually unilateral, they present as a uniform smooth scrotal swelling, which the patient has often had for some time. Discomfort due to a slow increase in size is a common complaint although most patients are simply worried about the swelling. On examination, it is possible to get above the swelling and it will trans-illuminate, unless there has been trauma or infection. It is often difficult to palpate the testis in large hydrocoeles. Radiological imaging is not mandatory, although often performed pre-operatively, unless there is reason to suspect an underlying testicular tumour. This is rare.

Treatment

Small hydrocoeles may be treated conservatively. Larger symptomatic hydrocoeles can be treated as a day case to surgically obliterate the tunical sac. It is inadvisable to aspirate hydrocoeles as they invariably recur and there is the potential to introduce infection and cause bleeding.

Patients should be warned that, following any type of scrotal surgery, complications are relatively common. They include infection, bleeding with the formation of a scrotal haematoma, and recurrence. The long-term outcome is, however, very good in the majority of cases.

Association

A developmental associate is the hydrocoele of the cord. In this condition, the processus vaginalis obliterates proximally and distally, leaving a fluid collection within the spermatic cord. If symptomatic this is relatively easy to excise.

Epididymal cysts

Also known as a spermatocoeles, these are cysts that are usually located in the head of the epididymis. The aetiology is unknown. They are picked up on routine medical examination or following self-examination. They are not typically painful.

They may become large enough to be misdiagnosed as a hydrocoele. The key difference is that the testis is palpable and *separate* from the swelling.

Small cysts, especially in men planning a family, should be managed expectantly. Large cysts can be excised as a day case via the scrotum. Complications are similar to patients having hydrocoele surgery. Recurrence is commoner.

Varicocoele

A varicocoele is due to dilatation of the pampiniform plexus of veins, which drain the testis. It is a common condition affecting up to 15% of the male population. Ninety per cent of cases occur on the left side. The exact aetiology is unclear. Several factors are thought to be involved, all leading to raised pressure in the testicular vein. These include incompetent venous valves, the long length of the testicular vein, and the nutcracker effect – compression of the left renal vein as it passes between the superior mesenteric artery and aorta.

Varicocoeles are traditionally thought to have a detrimental effect on the growth, development and function of the testis. The negative factors include increased testicular temperature, reflux of adrenal metabolites and intratesticular hyperperfusion injury.

Clinical features

Varicocoeles are usually asymptomatic and incidentally discovered by the patient, often after a warm shower. The patient may complain of a dragging sensation. The classic finding on examination is the feeling of a 'bag of worms' in the scrotum. It is best seen or felt with the patient in the standing position. A Valsalva manoeuvre will accentuate smaller varicocoeles (Table 6.2). It should empty when the patient is positioned supine. The testes should be examined, particularly in the adolescent, for retarded growth. An abdominal examination to rule out any masses completes the initial assessment.

Table 6.2 Varicocoele grading on examination.

Grade	Description
1	Small, palpable only with a Valsalva manoeuvre
2	Moderately sized, easily palpable without a Valsalva manoeuvre
3	Large, visible through the scrotal skin

Treatment

Small asymptomatic varicocoeles can be managed conservatively. Symptomatic cases or patients with retarded testicular growth require varicocoelectomy. This procedure can be carried out by radiological, open surgical or laparoscopic techniques. A 90% success rate should be quoted. Specific complications include recurrence, hydrocoele formation and testicular atrophy.

Associations

- Small testis: varicocoeles are associated with retarded testicular growth in the adolescent. This is an indication for surgical repair with catch-up growth seen in the affected testicle after treatment.
- Subfertility: this is contentious. Varicocoeles are commoner in infertile males (up to 40%) and semen quality following varicocoelectomy shows significant improvement. Against this association is a recent meta-analysis of data showing no overall improvement in conception rates post-varicocoele surgery. If a varicocoele is found in a patient with sub-fertility then it is best for advice to be sought from a urologist or fertility expert.
- Renal cancer: this is a rare association classically diagnosed following the discovery of a right hydrocoele. Tumour thrombus obstructs the inferior vena cava leading to obstruction of the right testicular vein and so causes the varicocoele. Because of this, it is common for patients presenting with varicocoele to have a renal ultrasound.

Epididymitis and orchitis

Epididymitis is inflammation of the epididymis, usually due to pathogenic micro-organisms. It occurs in two broad categories of patient – younger sexually active males (< 35 years) who have sexually transmitted infection (STI), and older males with prostatic problems, who have typical uropathogens such as *E. coli*. Patients with an abnormal urological tract – whether congenital or acquired – are also susceptible. Epididymitis is rare in the paediatric population and it is *important to exclude testicular torsion* first in these patients. It is worth pointing out the resurgence of mumps orchitis due to the decrease in the uptake of the MMR vaccine.

Clinical features

Epididymo-orchitis presents typically as gradual onset testicular pain and swelling, often with dysuria and fever. A past history of urinary tract infections, urethritis, urethral discharge, sexual activity, urethral catheterisation or urinary tract surgery is important to ascertain. Examination reveals a red swollen hemiscrotum and a tender enlarged epididymis and testis. The patient should undergo routine urological and abdominal examination specifically to look for an enlarged or tender prostate and a palpable bladder.

The presence of pyuria, bacteriuria, or a positive urine culture supports the diagnosis although urine cultures may be sterile in up to 90% of patients. A urethral swab is important in suspected STI. An ultrasound scan of the urological tract and testis is helpful in supporting the diagnosis and ruling out underlying causes. A flow rate and post-void residual should be done in the older male patient.

The main differential diagnosis is testicular torsion.

Treatment

- Bed rest and analgesia
- In the older male a prolonged course of a fluoroquinolone is recommended; e.g. Ciproxin 500 mg BD for 2–4 weeks (review at 2 weeks to assess response)
- In patients suspected of STI: Ofloxacin 400 mg BD for 2–4 weeks or Doxycycline 100 mg BD for 1 week
- Contact screening and treatment is advised.

Complications

Abscess formation, testicular infarction and atrophy, chronic epididymitis and infertility.

Torsion of testis

Torsion of the testis is due to twisting of the spermatic cord by rotation of a horizontally lying testis within a generous tunical attachment (bell clapper deformity). It is without doubt a surgical emergency as delay in untwisting of

Table 6.3 Differential diagnosis of testicular torsion.

Differential diagnosis	Discriminating factor
Epididymo-orchitis	Gradual onset, sexually active, urethral discharge *Rare in paediatric and adolescent*
Torted testicular appendage	Blue dot sign – unreliable
Idiopathic scrotal oedema	Dramatic erythema and swelling but the testis are usually non-tender and the patient comfortable
Ureteric colic	Radiated pain – testis non-tender

the cord results in ischaemic necrosis of the testis. The differential diagnosis of acute testicular pain and thus of testicular torsion is shown in Table 6.3.

Clinical features

Torsion presents as sudden onset severe testicular pain, often waking the patient from sleep. There may be a history of previous self-limiting acute scrotal pain. Nausea and vomiting may accompany the pain. The peak time of presentation is around puberty. It can, however, occur in any age group including the pre-natal group.

Examination reveals a patient in obvious discomfort. The consistent finding is a testis and spermatic cord that are exquisitely tender. More variable findings include a higher and transverse testicular lie and an absent cremasteric reflex. In later stages, the scrotum is erythematous and swollen. Atypical presentations are common. Patients may complain of only mild pain and some report lower abdominal pain alone. These patients should always have a careful testicular examination.

The diagnosis of testicular torsion is based on the history and examination. In equivocal cases urinalysis and colour Doppler ultrasound of the testis are helpful. Time is of the essence in these cases and urgent scrotal exploration is the best plan of action in most cases.

Treatment

■ Manual detorsion. This has been described – facing the patient and rotating the testis outward as in 'opening a book' to detort the testis. If this does not work then rotation in the opposite direction is suggested. It is very uncomfortable, but brings immediate relief if successful and may buy time in more remote areas. Even if successful, formal exploration and fixation should be carried out as soon as possible.

■ Surgical exploration, detorsion and bilateral fixation. Immediate surgical exploration is the definitive way of managing testicular torsion. Irreversible ischaemic injury to the testicle may begin as soon as 4 hours after occlusion of the cord. A midline scrotal incision is used. The affected testis is delivered, detorted and fixed to the scrotum with three non-absorbable sutures. The unaffected testis is also fixed as the anatomical variation of the bell clapper testis exists on both sides. If the torted testis is nonviable, it is removed and the contralateral testis is fixed. Insertion of a testicular prosthesis can be considered at a later date.

Torted testicular appendages

These are embryological cystic remnants which can tort and cause acute testicular pain. In many cases it is difficult to distinguish this condition from testicular torsion, so scrotal exploration is carried out. The torted appendage simply needs to be removed. There are no long-term consequences.

Summary

Most male patients who present to their GP with a 'lump in the testicle' are concerned about the possibility of malignancy. As pointed out, most conditions are benign and only those palpated *within* the testicle should be considered malignant. Once a patient has been examined and reassured that 'his lump' is benign, and the surgical route not chosen, then he should be encouraged to examine himself and get to know the benign lumps. If any changes or new lumps appear then he is advised to re-consult with his GP.

Key points

■ Scrotal and testicular pathology is a common trigger for consultations in general practice.

- A careful history and physical examination will confirm most lesions as benign without the need for further investigation.
- Lesions that cannot be palpated separate from the testis should be viewed as suspicious and referred for urgent assessment.
- Symptomatic patients or sub-fertile patients should be referred for further assessment.
- Emergency referral should be considered in all patients with acute testicular pain to avoid the potential disastrous consequences of missed testicular torsion.

Further reading and bibliography

European Associstion of Urology Guidelines (2008) http://www.uroweb.org/professional-resources/guidelines/; accessed June 2008.

Li, C. Y., Zaman, F. and Minhas, S. (2007) Testicular torsion and acute testicular pain. In: *Urological Emergencies in Hospital Medicine* (eds. I. S. Shergill, M. Arya, H. R. Patel and I. S. Gill), pp. 1–9. Quay Books, London.

CHAPTER 7

Ureteric colic

Hashim Uddin Ahmed, Paul Erotocritou, Shailesh Kulkarni, Peter Kraus and Matt Winkler

Case history

A 47-year-old gentleman presents to the community practice with a two-day history of right-sided abdominal pain which is increasing in severity. He is Asian and states he has been fasting during the Islamic religious month of Ramadhan. He complains that the pain is intermittent and is occasionally felt in the lower part of his abdomen. He feels nauseated but has not vomited and is opening his bowels. He has had no previous episodes. On examination he is not tender and has a normal temperature. Urine dipstix demonstrates blood 2+ and leucocytes 1+. The general practitioner arranges an urgent CT-KUB (non-contrast) at the local hospital, which demonstrates a 4 mm calculus in the right lower third ureter. Bloods, including urea, electrolytes and creatinine, and full blood count are requested and are all normal. The patient is managed in the community and empirical antibiotics are started due to the possibility of infection after a mid-stream urine specimen is sent for microbiology. Diclofenac (NSAID) 100 mg rectally once daily is also commenced as well as tamsulosin (an alpha-blocker) 400 mcg once daily. Twenty-four hours later he is pain-free, having passed the stone.

Introduction

Ureteric (renal) colic is a common condition, which often presents acutely. It is usually caused by calculi leading to obstruction of the ureter, but in approximately 15% of patients other causes are found, e.g. extrinsic compression due to pelvic or retroperitoneal fibrosis, intramural neoplasia or junctional abnormality such pelvi-ureteric junction (PUJ) obstruction. This chapter will focus on calculus renal colic, its assessment and subsequent management.

Traditionally, general practitioners (GPs) have admitted patients with this diagnosis directly to the urologist for confirmation of the diagnosis and subsequent management. However, the primary care physician can manage selected cases in the community with later out-patient follow-up so long as he or she is aware of appropriate diagnostic and management protocols and particularly the reasons for immediate referral to a specialist.

The incidence of urinary tract calculi in England and Wales is in the order of 28 per 100,000. In the main they are calcium stones (calcium oxalate, calcium phosphate, mixed calcium oxalate and phosphate), while 20% comprise the struvite (infective, triple phosphate, calcium/magnesium/ammonium phosphate) uric acid, and cystine groups. As ureteric colic is caused by obstruction of the urinary tract by calculi it is important to know the narrowest anatomical areas of the ureter, as this is where stones will impact. These are the PUJ; near the pelvic brim at the crossing of the iliac vessels; in women at the area where the broad ligament crosses over the ureter; and the narrowest area being the vesico-ureteric (VUJ) junction. The anatomical course of the ureters is illustrated in Figure 7.1.

History

Classically, ureteric colic presents with a sudden onset of acute loin or abdominal flank pain. The pain is colicky in nature and radiates across the abdomen to the groin and sometimes to the scrotum in men and the labia majora in women. Associated symptoms of nausea and vomiting are frequent while some mention intermittent frank haematuria. The differential diagnosis is large and includes appendicitis, pancreatitis, cholecystitis and, in women, salpingitis and tubal pathology. There are several reports of ruptured or leaking abdominal aneurysms presenting in a similar manner as ureteric colic and this should certainly be suspected in patients over 60 years of age with a first episode of loin pain and no previous history of renal stones. This differential should be kept in mind when taking a history (e.g. known gallstones, alcohol consumption, atherosclerosis) and examining patients (e.g. Murphy's sign, rebound/guarding) as well as ordering relevant investigations (e.g. chest radiograph for air under diaphragm). Mention should also be made of those who feign the symptoms of ureteric colic due to opiate dependency. One should be wary of this especially if a history of previous episodes treated in different distant hospitals is made.

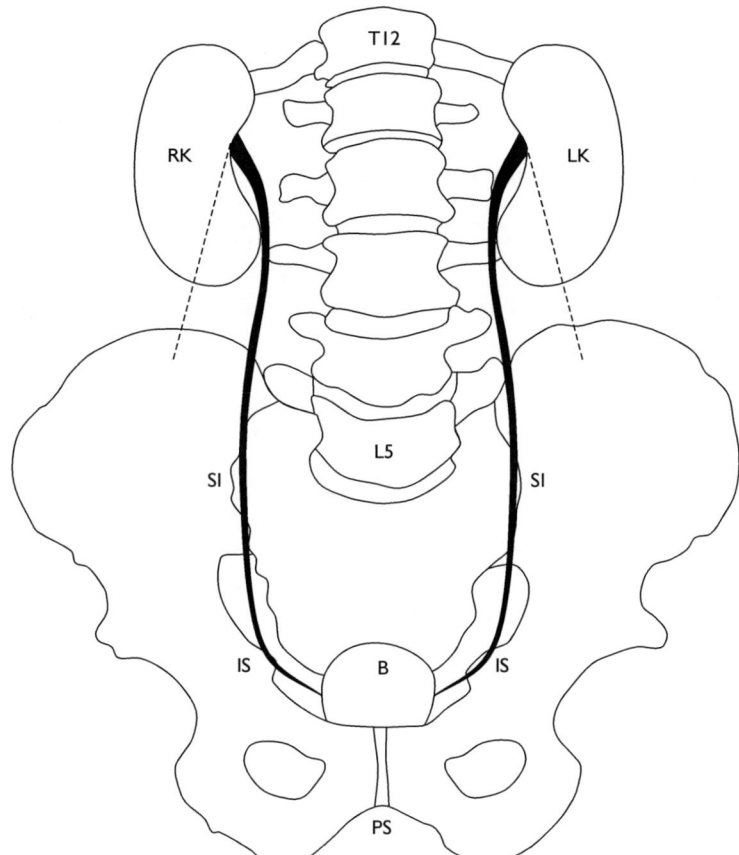

Figure 7.1 Anatomical course of ureters. RK = right kidney; LK = left kidney; T12/L5 = thoracic 12 and lumbar 5 vertebrae; dashed line = lateral outline of psoas major muscle; SI = sacroiliac joints; IS = ischial spine; PS = pubic symphysis; B= bladder. Each kidney lies obliquely alongside the psoas muscle. Right kidney lies half a vertebra lower, but both poles are at level of T12. Each ureter leaves the hilum of the kidney and courses just lateral to tips of vertebral transverse processes. Ureters cross the pelvic brim at the SI joint. They then tend towards the ischial spines laterally, and then medially towards the base of the bladder to enter the bladder obliquely through the bladder wall for 2–3 cm.

Examination

The patient is usually unable to remain still – this is a classic feature of colic as opposed to the 'still' peritonitic patient. If there is tachycardia and pyrexia this may indicate a concurrent urinary tract infection (UTI). Please note that an obstructed, infected kidney is a urological emergency and needs immediate hospital referral due to the risk of irreversible renal damage. Tachycardia and hypotension should alert the clinician to peritonitis from a ruptured viscus or aneurysm. Otherwise, examination reveals little else, with only a minority of patients exhibiting tenderness in the loin and at the site of the calculus.

Investigations

Urinalysis is mandatory since ureteric colic causes dipstix positive haematuria in over 90% of patients. A few patients have macroscopic haematuria. It is prudent to send a sample of urine for microscopy, culture and sensitivity to ascertain presence of bacteria.

A blood sample for full blood count, electrolytes, urea and creatinine, amylase, serum calcium, phosphate and urate are routinely sent. If appropriate, C-reactive protein and liver function tests may help if you suspect intraperitoneal pathology with beta-hCG mandatory in all pre-menopausal women.

A plain radiograph of the kidney-ureter-bladder (KUB) will identify radio-opaque calculi in about 80–90% of cases. A KUB also shows pelvic phleboliths and faecoliths which can cause diagnostic uncertainty to the untrained eye. Unless the stone is large, this test is generally of little value on its own and contrast studies such as an intravenous urogram are needed. Pure uric acid, xanthine and triamterene containing calculi are radiolucent. Cystine calculi are radiodense due to their sulphur content.

The intravenous urogram (IVU) is regarded as the gold standard for the diagnosis of renal and ureteric stones, although this has recently been challenged by other imaging modalities. The test is performed with intravenous injection of iodine-based contrast (e.g. Urograffin) after the plain KUB is taken, with subsequent serial radiographs usually at 20 minutes and post-micturition with delayed films if necessary where obstruction is demonstrated. This is apparent where there is delay in appearance of contrast material in the kidney and ureter. Comparison with control plain KUB will aid in identifying the location of the stone and its size.

One must be aware of the risks of sensitivity to intravenous contrast agents as well as excluding renal failure before performing this investigation. The latter will not only risk increased damage to the renal parenchyma, but also give a poor quality IVU. In diabetic patients taking metformin the iodine-based contrast reacts with the metformin causing a lactic acidosis; therefore the anti-glycaemic drug needs to be stopped 24–48 hours before and after the IVU.

In recent years, unenhanced helical computed tomography (commonly called CT-KUB) has been shown to be more sensitive and specific than IVU and ultrasound scan (USS) in detecting ureteric calculi. CT-KUB is useful in detecting radiodense as well as radiolucent calculi. Secondary signs of an obstructive process such as hydronephrosis as well as perinephric and periureteric stranding are readily identified. CT-KUB also provides significant alternative or additional diagnoses in 6–12% of cases. These advantages should be balanced against a two-fold increase in radiation exposure when compared to conventional three-film IVU, but as no contrast is used it is safe in those where IVU is contra-indicated. Furthermore, CT-KUB has now become the first line investigation in a number of centres.

Other investigative modalities have been studied. For example, the combination of a KUB and USS was found to be sensitive although not as specific for ureteric calculi as an IVU. Isotope renography (e.g. mercaptoacetyltriglycine [MAG-3]) has been used in conjunction with CT-KUB to assess anatomy as well as function: if there is no evidence of obstruction a CT-KUB is adequate, but isotope renography aids in distinguishing different degrees of obstruction when present. These findings, in conjunction with the clinical situation, size and site of the stone, identify those patients who would benefit from earlier intervention. More recently, magnetic resonance imaging has been evaluated and recent studies have shown it to have certain advantages over CT-KUB, especially in detecting obstruction. It is of particular importance in evaluating renal colic in pregnant women, as there is no radiation exposure.

We recommend the GP should arrange a CT-KUB within one week of presentation to confirm the diagnosis of ureteric colic.

Management and discussion

This involves analgesia, anti-emetics and adequate hydration. Much debate has centred on whether non-steroidal anti-inflammatory drugs (NSAIDs) or opiate-based analgesia should be used. Recent meta-analysis of trials which compared these two groups reached the conclusion that NSAIDs are more effective in pain relief, require less rescue medication, induce fewer side effects (such as nausea and vomiting), and are useful in stone expulsion by reducing ureteric inflammation. If opiates are to be used, the recommendation is for pethidine to be avoided, as it causes more nausea and vomiting. We suggest that first-line analgesia should consist of 100 mg Diclofenac rectally once daily (or 75 mg by intramuscular injection). If there are any contraindications to NSAIDs, intramuscular pethidine or oral tramadol are alternatives in conjunction with an anti-emetic if necessary. The patient should be reassessed by the GP in 2 to 3 hours, by telephone if convenient, to check the response to analgesia. The patient should be advised to maintain normal hydration.

The discovery of alpha-1 adrenergic receptors in the distal ureter led to studies looking at tamsulosin, a selective alpha-1 antagonist normally used in the treatment of benign prostatic hyperplasia to relax prostatic smooth muscle. It has been shown that tamsulosin 400 mcg once daily aids in the early expulsion of distal small ureteric stones, hence reducing the need for endoscopic intervention, hospitalisation and analgesic use.

Patients with infection and obstructing calculus need to be referred urgently to a urologist (due to risk of irreversible renal damage) and treated vigorously with intravenous fluids and empirical broad-spectrum antibiotics in the first instance. If renal ultrasound scan confirms the presence of hydronephrosis urgent renal decompression with a nephrostomy or retrograde stent is mandatory to prevent irreversible renal damage and septicaemia. Nephrostomy is usually opted for, as these patients tend to be septic and therefore the avoidance of a general anaesthetic is usually advocated if possible. Uroseptic patients tend to be very unwell and therefore need intensive clinical monitoring, ideally with management in a high dependency unit.

Patients with stones causing significant obstruction and intractable pain will again need urological referral, with probable ureteric stenting pending definitive treatment. This can have a failure rate of up to 20% and require subsequent percutaneous drainage and antegrade stenting via a nephrostomy. Some urologists, however, would institute definitive treatment with ureteroscopic stone fragmentation and extraction. This may be followed by insertion of a temporary ureteric stent if there is significant inflammation or damage to the ureter.

Reasons for urgent hospital referral in patients with renal colic (including those mentioned above) are:

- Ureteric colic associated with infection (suggested by fever)
- Intractable pain unresponsive to prescribed analgesia
- Renal failure
- Solitary kidney
- Uncertain of diagnosis (it is uncommon for a patient >60 years of age to present with a first episode of ureteric colic – must exclude leaking abdominal aortic aneurysm in this group)
- Inability to arrange early investigation to confirm diagnosis

If a calculus is confirmed on investigation and the patient managed at home, he or she should be encouraged to sieve the urine for stones and a urological out-patient appointment should be arranged, preferably within two weeks.

Definitive treatment

Definitive treatment of the ureteric calculus is dependent on its size and site. Calculi less than 4 mm in size are likely to pass spontaneously in the majority of cases (80%). In patients with stones of this size, who have good pain control and have no evidence of infection, primary care management is possible with follow-up imaging needed after 2–3 weeks. The probability of spontaneous passage of stones is not only dependent on size, but also on site. Overall spontaneous ureteral stone passage rate is:

- Proximal ureter   25%
- Mid-ureter   45%
- Distal ureter   70%

Patients should be encouraged to sieve urine in order to recover calculi as this allows chemical analysis of the stone, especially in the setting of recurrent stone formation. As has been suggested, not all patients with ureteric colic need hospital admission. Hospital admission is necessary when pain is not controlled with oral analgesics; in the presence of anuria and risk of renal failure (patients with an obstructing calculus in a solitary kidney or rarely, bilateral obstruction); or in the presence of concomitant infection. These are also obvious indications for intervention.

Proximal ureteric non-obstructing stones can be treated by extra-corporeal shock wave lithotripsy (ESWL) with stone free rates above 80%. Contraindications to ESWL are pregnancy, uncontrolled coagulopathy, uncontrolled hypertension and febrile urinary tract infection. Endoscopic treatment is reserved for large (>1 cm) stones, multiple stones, hard stones (e.g. cystine) or impacted stones causing significant obstruction.

Mid-ureteric calculi can either be treated with ESWL or ureteroscopy. Although good results have been obtained with ESWL, localisation of the stone radiographically may be difficult in this region due to the pelvic bones. Flexible ureteroscopes are useful to access the stones in this area.

Lower ureteric calculi can be treated successfully with ureteroscopy under general anaesthesia as a day case procedure. Rarely, a ureteric stent may need to be inserted at the end of the procedure where there is traumatic extraction or uncertainty about ureteric injury. ESWL has satisfactory results as a first line treatment for smaller calculi (<1 cm) where facilities are available.

Investigation and prevention of further stones

The underlying abnormality predisposing to stone formation remains after spontaneous stone passage or surgical stone removal, and therefore identifiable causes in calcium metabolism (hyperparathyroidism, sarcoidosis) or oxalate metabolism (primary oxaluria) need to be ascertained in recurrent stone formers and treated appropriately. Similarly, uric acid and cystine stone formers will need appropriate therapy for the underlying problem. Generally, a metabolic stone screen is not performed following a single episode of ureteric colic. However, in those patients with recurrent or bilateral stones, paediatric stone formers and those with a family history of renal stones a metabolic stone screen is performed in order to identify a cause. This consists of serum calcium, phosphate, urate and creatinine levels as well as 24 hour urinary pH and volume and 24 hour urine levels of calcium, oxalate, urate, phosphate, magnesium, sodium and creatinine, and a urine spot test for cystine.

Adequate fluid intake to maintain a urine output in the region of 3 litres for an average sized person per day reduces stone recurrence: this is the main guidance provided to the majority of patients to prevent recurrence of idiopathic urinary tract calculi.

Specific dietary modifications

Patients should eat a mixed balanced diet with contributions from all food groups. There is general advice that could be given to patients:

- *Fruits, vegetables and fibres*: should be encouraged because of the beneficial effects of fibre and the ability of vegetables to alkinise the urine.
- *Oxalate*: excessive intake of oxalate-rich products should be avoided to prevent an oxalate load. This is important in patients in shown to have a high oxalate excretion. Rhubarb, spinach, cocoa, tea leaves (but not coffee) and nuts have a high content of oxalate.
- *Animal protein*: avoid excessive amounts (recommended intake limited to 0.8–1 g/kg body weight). Excess gives rise to several hypocitraturia, low pH, hyperoxaluria and hyperuricosuria, and increased resorption of bone increases urinary calcium. These promote stone formation.
- *Calcium*: should *not* be restricted. In fact, it has been suggested that calcium restriction may actually promote stone formation.
- *Sodium*: high consumption causes calcium excretion and reduced urine citrate. Therefore, risk of forming sodium urate crystals is increased. The combined restriction of sodium and animal protein in a randomised study

resulted in a reduced rate of calcium stone formation. The daily sodium intake should not exceed 3 g.

- *Urate*: in patients with hyperuricosuric calcium oxalate stone disease and uric acid stone disease urate intake should be restricted (urate not to exceed 500 mg/day). Examples of food rich in urate include: calf thymus, liver, kidneys, poultry skin, herring with skin, sardines, anchovies, sprats.

Key points

- Uncomplicated calculus related ureteric colic can be managed in the community.
- The GP should exclude other surgical diagnosis and be particularly wary of leaking abdominal aortic aneurysms in patients over 60 years of age, which may mimic the pain of ureteric colic
- Appropriate imaging such as plain KUB, IVU, USS or preferably a CT-KUB without contrast should be requested by the GP (and performed within a week) to confirm the diagnosis
- A ureteric stone associated with fever should be referred immediately to the urologist, as an obstructed, infected kidney is a urological emergency.
- NSAIDs (ideally Diclofenac 100 mg rectally) are the most appropriate analgesic agent to use and with adequate hydration most stones will pass spontaneously.
- The use of tamsulosin (400 mcg once daily) as an adjunct in the conservative management of ureteric calculi (particularly those in the distal one third of the ureter) has been proven effective.

Further reading and bibliography

Ahmed, H., Khan, A., Bafaloukas, N. and Buchholz, N. (2007) Diagnosis and management of renal (ureteric) colic. In: *Urological Emergencies in Hospital Medicine* (eds. I. S. Shergill, M. Arya, H. R. Patel and I. S. Gill), pp. 17–26. Quay Books, London.

Ahmad, N. A., Ather, M. H. and Rees, J. (2003) Incidental diagnoses of diseases on un-enhanced helical tomography performed for ureteric colic. *BMC Urol.*, **3**, 2.

European Association of Urology Guidelines (2008) http://www.uroweb.org/professional-resources/guidelines/; accessed June 2008.

Greenwell, T. J., Woodhams, S., Denton, E. R., MacKenzie, A., Rankin, S. C. and Popert, R. (2000) One year's clinical experience with unenhanced spiral computed tomography for the assessment of acute loin pain suggestive of renal colic. *BJU International*, **85**, 632–6.

Holdgate, A. and Pollack, T. (2005) Nonsteroidal anti-inflammatory drugs (NSAIDs) vs opioids for acute renal colic. *Cochrane Database Syst. Rev.*, **18**(2), CD004137.

Morris, S. B., Hampson, S. J., Gordon, E. M., Shearer, R. J. and Woodhouse, C. R. (1995) Should all patients with ureteric colic be admitted? *Ann. R. Coll. Surg.*, **77**, 450–2.

CHAPTER 8

Benign and malignant skin disorders of the external genitalia

Iaisha Ali, Mohamed Hammadeh, Shailesh Kulkarni, Navroop Shergill and Asif Muneer

Benign non-infectious conditions

Psoriasis

This is a common skin condition that can affect the genitalia. Lesions usually present as erythematous patches or plaques with a scaly surface that are usually non-itchy. The perineum and natal cleft are also commonly affected. Genital skin can be the sole site of disease; however, examination of the body, scalp and nails can be helpful as this may reveal more lesions. Typical sites to examine on the body that may guide diagnosis are the extensor surfaces of elbows, knees and umbilicus.

The diagnosis can often be made on clinical grounds, but a biopsy may be required in some cases.

Treatment options include topical steroid, weak coal tar preparations and vitamin D analogues. Topical calcineurin inhibitors have also been used for genital psoriasis with some success, although this is an unlicensed use. Super-added fungal or bacterial infection can be a problem in genital psoriasis and therefore steroid preparation containing antifungal and/or antibiotic additives can help prevent exacerbation if infection is suspected.

Eczema and lichen simplex

Atopic eczema is a form of 'allergic' eczema that is associated with other forms of allergic tendency such as asthma and hayfever. Localised atopic eczema can develop at genital sites such as the scrotum and the base of the penis. Pruritis is the key symptom in eczema and this can acutely result in redness and excoriation caused by scratching. Secondary bacterial infection can commonly develop in patches of eczema resulting in crusting and weeping exudation. Lesions should be swabbed if infection is suspected.

Topical steroids are the mainstay of treatment for eczema. Because of the risk of secondary infection, treatment with a combination corticosteroid and antibacterial/ antifungal cream is usually quite effective. If more severe infection is present, a course of oral antibiotics may be required.

Lichen simplex is a form of eczema that results from chronic itching. This causes a uniform thickening of the skin described as lichenification. A careful history may identify a potential irritant, although habit can play a significant part in this condition. Skin changes of can be reversed through regular moisturisation, avoidance of irritants and habit reversal techniques aimed to help break the 'itch–scratch' cycle.

Seborrhoeic forms of eczema can also affect the genital region. Lesions may appear as red, moist patches without much scaling. Treatment with an antifungal cream can relieve symptoms. Patients should be advised to avoid clothing that may be occlusive and promote moisture retention. More resistant cases may require a course of oral anti-fungal medication.

Contact allergy

Local application of topical pharmaceuticals or creams can result in sensitisation to chemical elements or preservatives within the topical agent. Contact allergy is more frequently seen in patients with a history of inflammatory skin disease such as eczema. The main symptoms are burning and pruritis. A careful history to identify topical agents applied to the area is essential. Patch testing can help verify the diagnosis. Lubricants, spermicides, deodorants and latex condoms are the most commonly found causative agents for genital allergy.

Fixed drug eruption

The genital areas and acral sites are the most common for fixed drug eruptions. Twenty per cent of fixed drug eruptions involve the genitalia. This is a form of drug allergy that manifests as a localised skin eruption that does not involve any physical contact with the causative agent. There is usually a latency period of between 24 and 48 hours from taking the drug and the development of localised erythema that can progress to vesiculation. Subsequent exposure to the causative agent can result in an enhanced reaction at the same site.

The most frequent agents implicated in fixed drug eruption include trimethoprim, tetracyclines, sulphadiazines, acetaminophen and metronidazole. Provocation testing or specialised patch testing can be performed to confirm diagnosis.

Lichen sclerosus (balanitis xerotica obliterans)

Lichen sclerosus (LS) is a chronic sclerosing inflammatory dermatosis. Most reported cases of LS (83%) involve the genitalia. Genital involvement in men is traditionally known as balanitis xerotica obliterans (BXO) (Figure 8.1). A more accurate term is male genital or penile LS. It is more commonly seen in middle aged men, although the age range for presentation is wide and includes young children and adolescents.

The cause of LS is largely unknown and thought to involve multiple factors. There is some evidence to suggest an autoimmune aetiology.

LS can present with a variety of symptoms: non-specific irritation, itching, burning and dyspareunia. Later signs include discomfort on urination

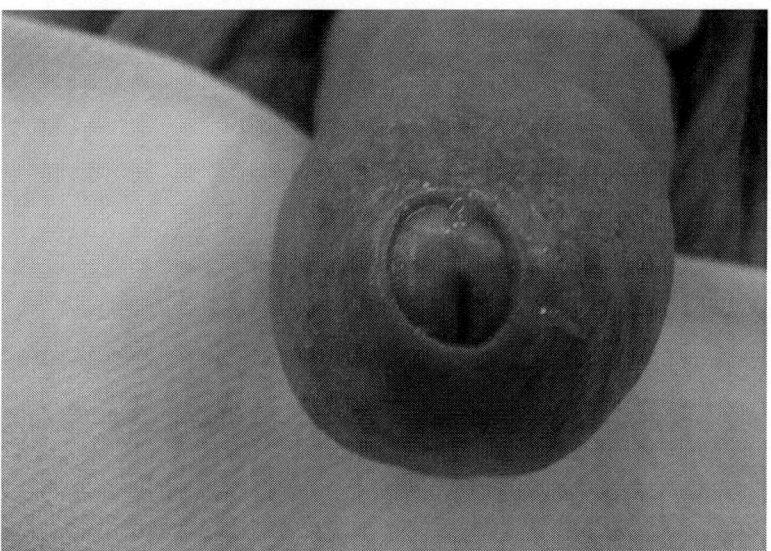

Figure 8.1 A typical case of balanitis xerotica obliterans showing phimosis and tight scarred foreskin.

and narrowing of the urinary stream. Lesions may appear as lilac, atrophic pale patches or plaques. Bullae, erosions and ulceration may also be seen. More severe cases can present with phimosis, paraphimosis (with a thickened, scarred prepuce) and even urinary retention and renal failure due to the development of urethral stricture, as the disease process can involve the urethra.

Extragenital involvement in LS is common and has been reported with a frequency of 17%. At extragenital sites, LS can appear as patches or plaques of erythema or ivory white atrophic scarring.

The differential diagnosis in genital LS includes lichen planus. A biopsy should be performed to confirm diagnosis. This should be done urgently if there are signs of erosion or verrucous change due to the risk of developing squamous cell cancer in 6% of cases.

Treatment is with ultra-potent corticosteroid under supervision. Other agents that have been used include topical calcineurin inhibitors and oral retinoids. However, circumcision is often required when the prepuce is involved. As LS is a chronic and progressive condition long term follow up is recommended.

Lichen planus

This is a common condition that can affect the skin and mucosal surfaces. Cutaneous lesions can appear in a wide variety of forms but the typical cutaneous presentation is of intensely itchy, violaceous papules, patches or plaques. Common sites include the extensor surface of the wrist and the ankles. A linear streaking pattern may be seen in the mouth known as Wickham's striae.

In genital disease, typically, an annular configuration of papules is seen on the glans. Less commonly, linear white striae, similar to the lesions on the buccal mucosa can be seen on male genitalia. Erosive forms can also develop on mucosal sites resulting in ulceration.

Medical treatment is with potent topical steroid. Circumcision may be necessary. Oral steroids or retinoids may be required for generalised disease.

Zoon's balanitis

Plasma cell balanitis (PCB) was described by a Dutch dermatologist called Zoon in 1954. It is a condition that mainly affects uncircumcised middle aged and elderly men. Although benign, it is vital to distinguish this from penile Bowen's disease (Erythroplasia of Queyrat).

PCB presents as well-demarcated shiny, bright red or brownish patches that involve the glans and prepuce (often in opposed distribution; the so-called 'kissing lesion'). The etiology of PCB is unknown. It has been proposed that friction, trauma, heat, poor hygiene, chronic infection with *Mycobacterium smegmatis*, a reactive response to an unknown exogenous or infectious agent, an immediate hypersensitivity response mediated by immunoglobulin E class antibodies, and hypospadias may be predisposing or inciting agents. There is no evidence of human papilloma virus infection in PCB. The diagnosis can be established clinically; however, biopsy is often necessary for confirmation. The characteristic histopathologic findings include epidermal orthokeratosis and atrophy with focal vacuolar change of the basal layer and hyalinisation of the papillary and superficial reticular dermis. A superficial perivascular lymphocytic inflammatory infiltrate is frequently present.

Circumcision is recommended. CO_2 laser has also been applied as an alternative to circumcision.

Reiter's syndrome and circinate balanitis

Reiter's syndrome is an episode of peripheral arthritis and urethritis. It is frequently accompanied by circinate balanitis, conjunctivitis and keratoderma blennorrhagicum. Circinate balanitis can be observed in 12–70% of cases of Reiter's syndrome. A large number of pathogenic organisms can act as a trigger for Reiter's. The disease occurs primarily in genetically predisposed individuals, particularly those with HLA-B27, and is most commonly triggered by bacterial infectious agents. *C. trachomatis* is responsible for triggering most cases. Enteric infection with *Yersinia, Salmonella, Shigella* and *Campylobacter* species are also common infectious triggers for Reiter's syndrome. The exact pathogenetic mechanisms involved in induction of this condition are unknown. Up to 90% of patients are HLA-B27 positive.

Behcet disease

This is defined as the presence of recurrent oral ulceration and two minor criteria, which include genital ulceration, eye pathology, pseudofolliculitis and positive pathergy.

On the genital areas, ulcers can be present on the glans, scrotum or perianal skin. Ulcers are deep, sharply defined, painful and heal with atrophic scarring. Histology from the ulcers in non-specific and does not aid diagnosis. There is an association with HLA-B51, B27 and –B12. Differential diagnosis would include Crohn's or drug-induced ulceration.

Angiokeratomas

These appear as blue papules on the scrotal skin or penile shaft. Numbers can increase with time. Bleeding can be a problem. They can be mistaken for bacillary angiomatosis or Kaposi's sarcoma.

Tyson's gland (gland of Fordyce)

Prominent sebaceous glands, also called Tyson's gland or gland of Fordyce are normal variants. They can be present on the scrotal skin and penile shaft. Patients may be concerned about the appearance of their skin and reassurance is required.

Pearly penile papules

These occur in 15–20% of men. They are small 1-2 mm pale or flesh coloured papules with a smooth round surface. They are usually found in a linear distribution around the coronal margin of the glans and can be mistaken for warts. Histology is of angiofibroma. Treatment is not required; however, cryotherapy can be effective if necessary for cosmesis.

Premalignant conditions

Erythroplasia of Queyrat and Bowen's disease

Erythroplasia of Queyrat was originally described by Tarnovsky in 1891. It arises from the squamous epithelial cells of the glans penis or inner lining of the prepuce. It is seen almost exclusively in uncircumcised men and represents an *in situ* form of squamous cell carcinoma on the glans and prepuce (Figure 8.2). Progression to invasive carcinoma may occur after a variable period of time.

It presents as a red shiny patch which can be eroded. It is associated with oncogenic HPV types. Biopsy is essential.

Medical treatment with topical 5-flourouracil cream has been shown to be effective in some cases. There have been case reports of success with topical Imiquimod. Photodynamic therapy is also an option.

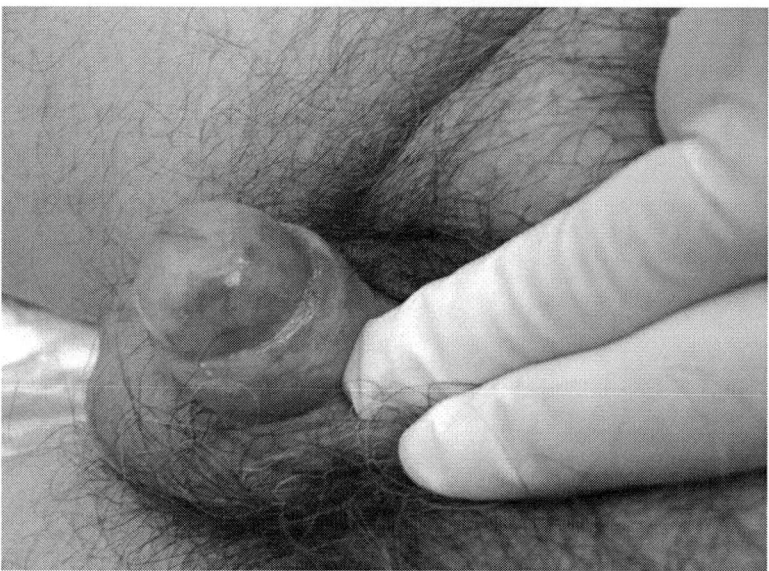

Figure 8.2 Erythroplasia of Queyrat (carcinoma *in situ* of the glans and inner prepuce).

Surgical treatments include curettage and cautery, electrodessication, CO_2 laser ablation and Mohs micrographic surgery.

Early detection can ensure a cure rate of up to 90%. Although this condition is significantly more frequent in uncircumcised men, adult circumcision does not seen to improve prognosis.

Bowen's disease is squamous cell carcinoma *in situ* of the penile shaft and scrotum (c.f. Erythroplasia of Queyrat, which is the same condition of the glans or inner prepuce). It presents as a thickened gray–white plaque in those over 35 years. It has a greater chance of progression to invasive carcinoma than Erythroplasia of Queyrat. Management options are similar.

Bowenoid papulosis

This is histologically similar to Bowen's disease, but generally has a benign course. It presents as multiple rather than solitary, reddish to brown pigmented lesions (Figure 8.3). The condition is induced by HPV infection with HPV types 16 and 18 most commonly implicated. Other types involved include types 31, 32, 34, 39, 42, 48, 51–54. Swabbing the lesional area with acetic acid 5% can help delineate the extent of the lesion.

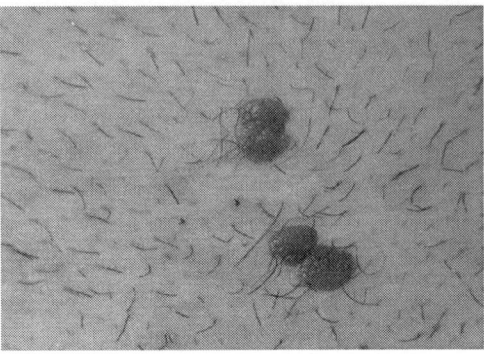

Figure 8.3 Bowenoid papulosis.

Paget's disease

Extramammary Paget's disease (EPD) has a predilection for areas with a high density of apocrine glands. Anogenital involvement with extramammary Paget's is relatively frequent. The relationship between EPD and malignancy is not completely understood. Three patterns of EPD have been identified: an intra-epithelial *in situ* form without associated cancer; an epithelial form with associated adnexal cancer; EPD associated with visceral malignancy. An intensive examination with respect to visceral malignancy and anogenital cancer is required although 50% of cases do not reveal any associated cancer.

Kaposi's sarcoma

This is most commonly seen in the context of HIV. It has a predilection for the mucosa and can occur in the form of patch, papular and nodular and haemorrhagic forms. Phimosis can occur. Treatment with highly active retro-viral therapy can lead to complete resolution of localised cutaneous Kaposi's sarcoma.

Infections

Pubic lice

Pediculosis pubis or crabs is caused by an infestation with a louse (*Phthirus pubis*). They are spread usually through sexual contact. They appear as 1–2 mm tan brown attachments to the hair shaft. A central dark area may be seen in the body of the louse after feeding. Patients develop itching several weeks after infestations. Lice can survive off the human body for up to 24 hours. Nits or eggs may be attached to the hair, typically as 1 mm solid concretions better seen with magnification. Blue macules may appear on the groin at the site of bites.

Patients typically present with genital itching in the absence of visible lesions. The infestations readily responds to permethrin or lindane application. If untreated, the infestation may spread to the axillary hairs and even the eyelids. The nits can be removed with a fine-toothed comb.

Tinea cruris

Tinea cruris is a relatively common problem. Typically, patients complaining of a rash present for several weeks or months in the groin. Most patients have typically tried several over the counter creams, powder, or sprays before presenting to a doctor. Inciting factors include obesity and excessive heat and humidity. On examination, diffuse bilateral erythema and scaling along the inguinal folds with a raised scaly border typical of tinea infection is usually present. The eruption may extend along the perineum up the gluteal cleft. Involvement of the scrotum is distinctly uncommon and another diagnosis should be considered with extensive scrotal involvement. Most tinea cruris are caused by fungi like *Trichophytan rubrum* (for treatment refer to section on candidiasis below).

Candidiasis

Candidiasis also occurs in the inguinal folds. The eruption is erythematous and scaly but usually without a raised border. Both tinea cruris and candidiasis readily respond to topical antifungal treatment such miconazole, ketoconazole or terbinafine.

Removing environmental factors such as heat, sweat, and obesity are important to prevent reinfection.

Erythrasma

Erythrasma is an uncommon bacterial infection caused by *Corynebacterium minisutum* that presents with diffuse thin red patches along the inguinal folds.

Unlike tinea cruris, no raised border or central clearing is noted. Diagnosis can be aided by a Wood's light in which the infection shines a coral pink fluorescent colour. Treatment is easily accomplished with topical or oral antibiotics such as erythromycin or clindamycin.

Herpes simplex (HSV)

HSV infection is the most common cause of genital ulcers in developed countries. Most cases of genital herpes are due to HSV-2. HSV is a lipid-enveloped DNA virus that predominantly infects mucosal or cutaneous surfaces. The virus replicates at the site of infection and then travels retrogradely via sensory nerves to the dorsal root ganglion, where latency is established. Multiple mechanisms are involved in reactivation of the virus, including altered immunity, tissue damage, stress, and/or ultraviolet light exposure. During reactivation, the virus begins replicating at or around the site of initial exposure. Dissemination to extracutaneous sites may occur, depending on the host immune response.

HSV-2 has a predilection for the anogenital region, whereas HSV-1 predominantly affects orolabial skin and mucosa. HSV transmission occurs through viral shedding from active lesions in symptomatic individuals, as well as through viral shedding from asymptomatic individuals with a history of infection.

Symptomatic primary genital herpes manifests within three weeks of initial exposure. Males typically experience regional pain and an eruption characterised by clustered papulovesicles. Associated herpetic urethritis may manifest with dysuria and urethral discharge. Over 2–3 weeks, painful skin lesions progress to pustules and erosions or ulcerations. Lesions heal with crusting. Regional lymphadenopathy and systemic constitutional symptoms may be present.

The most common location in males is the penis, the glans, or the shaft; however, any part of the anogenital region may be affected. Regional nongenital skin, such as that of the thigh, buttocks or pubic area, is also a common site of recurrent genital HSV. Many individuals experience a neuropathic prodrome, such as itching, tingling or burning, prior to the onset of lesions.

Isolation of the herpes virus in cell culture is the most definitive diagnostic test. Culture of early lesions, such as that of a vesicle or moist ulcer, has the highest diagnostic yield. Tzanck smear may also be useful and can yield results more quickly than other tests. However, identification of the multinucleated epithelial cells with intranuclear inclusions is sometimes difficult and does not distinguish HSV infection from infection from other herpesviruses. PCR testing is available through reference laboratories.

Treatment involves a 10 day course of oral acyclovir.

Syphilis

Syphilitic infection is acquired through sexual contact with an infected individual. The spirochete organism *Treponema pallidum* is the causative agent.

The organism enters through the skin and/or mucous membranes, and manifestations are noted after a 2–4 week incubation.

Syphilis infection typically involves three distinct clinical stages. The primary lesion, known as a chancre, develops at the site of inoculation. The next stage, secondary syphilis, results in various clinical manifestations, primarily in the skin and mucous membranes. Lesions in both the first and second stages contain numerous treponemal organisms and are consequently contagious. Following the second stage is a period of latency. The third stage, known as tertiary syphilis, is characterised by cardiovascular and/or central nervous system involvement. Tertiary syphilis is rare and develops in approximately one third of untreated infected individuals.

Primary syphilis presents as a discrete painless penile ulcer (chancre). The lesion is usually located on the glans, foreskin or scrotum. Up to 5% may present in extragenital locations. Anorectal lesions are common in infected homosexual males and can present clinically as anal fissures. Nontender inguinal lymphadenopathy may be present. The chancre spontaneously resolves within 3–6 weeks.

The second stage of syphilis occurs 6–8 weeks after developing the chancre. The classic presentation is of a widespread macular and papular eruption involving the palms and soles, the oral mucosa may also be involved. The clinical manifestations of secondary syphilis are greatly variable.

The diagnostic criterion standard for primary syphilis is the demonstration of the spirochete in scrapings from a syphilitic lesion with dark-field microscopy. Non-treponemal antibody tests, such as venereal disease research laboratory (VDRL), are used as screening tests.

Treatment with penicillin G is the recommended treatment for primary, secondary and latent syphilis.

Balanoposthitis

Defined as the inflammation of the foreskin and glans in uncircumcised males, balanoposthitis occurs over a wide age range and may have any of multiple bacterial or fungal origins or be caused by contact dermatitides. Complex infections have been well documented, often from a poorly retractile foreskin and poor hygiene that leads to colonisation and overgrowth. Treatment focuses on clearing the acute infection and preventing recurrent inflammation/infection through improved hygiene. Although not as necessary as in the past, circumcision may be considered for refractory or recurrent balanoposthitis. Although multiple organisms have been incriminated as causative agents, the patient is empirically treated without obtaining specific organism aetiology in most cases. The multicausal origin of balanoposthitis has been emphasised by the fact that infectious, mechanical/traumatic mechanisms or contact dermatitides are identified in 67% of patients with balanoposthitis. In one third of patients, a specific cause cannot be established even after clinical examination and microbiologic and serologic tests are performed. Candidal infection appears to be the most common cause of disease. Older men often have other aetiologies, including intertrigo, irritant dermatitides, or other fungal infections. Organisms that have been identified include *Bacteroides, Gardnerella* and *Candida* species and beta-haemolytic streptococci.

It has been proposed that candidal balanitis/balanoposthitis is the most frequent mycotic infection of the penis, although in general fungal infections of the penis are rare. Some investigators have identified *Candida* species as accounting for 30% of the causative organisms, and beta-hemolytic streptococci for 13%. Others have detected the following infectious agents as a cause: *Candida* species in 50%, *Streptococcus* species in 25%, and no growth in 13%, with the remaining not being tested.

Treatment involves topical antibiotics (e.g. metronidazole cream, clotrimazole cream, fucidin cream) or low-potency steroid creams for contact dermatitides. Proper hygiene with frequent washing and drying of the prepuce is an essential preventive measure.

Molluscum contagiosum

These are caused by a DNA pox virus infection and look like small, flesh-coloured papules with umbilicated centres. Multiple and giant lesions can occur with HIV infection or other forms of immunosuppression. Lesions usually regress spontaneously. Mollusca can be treated with cryotherapy or curettage and cautery. Patients should be screened for sexually transmitted infection if relevant.

Key points

- Non-healing or persistent areas of ulceration must have a biopsy to exclude malignancy.

- Common inflammatory skin diseases such as eczema and psoriasis can involve the genitalia; therefore it is important to examine all the skin.
- Remember to take swabs from lesion as super-added infection can complicate the clinical picture.
- Combined steroid, antifungal and antibiotic ointments are a suitable first line treatment for inflammatory genital dermatoses, but if lesions are unresponsive a biopsy is required to confirm diagnosis.
- Benign genital lesions are common and often reassurance to the patient is the only action required.

Further reading and bibliography

Link, R. E. (2007) Cutaneous diseases of the external genitalia. In: *Campbell-Walsh Urology*, 9th edn (eds. A. J. Wein, L. R. Kavoussi, A. C. Novick, A. W. Partin and C. A. Peters), pp. 405–35. Saunders Elsevier, Philadelphia, PA.

CHAPTER 9

Lower urinary tract symptoms and benign prostatic hyperplasia

Neil Barber and Gordon Mackay

Case history

A 63-year-old man presents to the surgery with a long history of ever-slowing stream of urine and some urinary frequency. More recently he has developed worsening urgency of micturition, which is having a significant effect upon his confidence at work and in undertaking long journeys. Furthermore, having previously got up usually once at night to pass urine, he now voids two or three times each night, which has resulted in a deleterious effect upon his quality of sleep and he is therefore feeling increasingly exhausted.

Introduction

This patient represents not only an individual part of the 60% of men of his age who will describe significant lower urinary tract symptoms (LUTS) on questioning, but also the 25% who will actually seek medical advice regarding them. It is characteristic that it is those symptoms relating to the storage of urine (storage symptoms = urinary frequency, urgency, urge incontinence and nocturia) that brings men to their GP as they are often considered of most bother and therefore have greatest effect upon quality of life. As in this case, there may be a longer history of voiding or 'obstructive' symptoms (poor stream, hesitancy in the initiation of the void and sensation of poor bladder emptying), although often not considered too bothersome, and the patient therefore presents with a 'mixed picture' of LUTS.

How to assess a man with bothersome LUTS in the first instance

History

As always, a thorough medical history is very important and can be supplemented by the use of a validated questionnaire such as the International Prostate Symptom Score (IPSS), which includes a quality of life score (Table 9.1). It is also important to determine whether there has been any history of frank haematuria or episodes of urosepsis or urogenital infections, as positive responses will require a different approach in terms of investigation.

It is also important to discover or otherwise any co-existing or previous medical conditions that may influence urinary tract function or indeed dysfunction. This particularly relates to regular medications prescribed for other conditions, e.g. alpha-blockers, diuretics and drugs with anti-cholinergic side effects, any neurological diseases or events, e.g. recent CVA, Parkinson's disease and previous pelvic or uro-genital surgery.

Finally, a thorough appreciation of the patient's drinking and voiding habit is made, preferably using a voiding diary or frequency–volume chart in combination with a record of the type of beverage imbibed.

Examination

A full abdominal examination and palpation of the prostate is necessary to exclude frank malignancy, chronic retention (i.e. painless, palpable bladder) and provide some idea as to the size of the prostate. Estimating the volume of the prostate is not only inaccurate, but also not hugely useful. As we shall see, in terms of influencing management, it is simply important to note if the prostate feels 'enlarged' or not. In that sense the digital rectal examination (DRE) is very accurate.

Table 9.1 The IPSS score with supplementary quality of life question. The IPSS scores seven questions on a scale from 0 to 5. Mild LUTS is defined as a score of 0–7, moderate LUTS scores 8–19, and severe LUTS scores 20–35. The quality of life question is scored from 0–6.

Over the past month, how often have you:	Not at all	Less than 1 time in 5	Less than half the time	About half the time	More than half the time	Almost always
1. ...had a sensation of not emptying your bladder completely after you finished urinating?	0	1	2	3	4	5
2. ...had to urinate again less than two hours after you finished urinating?	0	1	2	3	4	5
3. ...stopped and started again several times when you urinated?	0	1	2	3	4	5
4. ...found it difficult to postpone urination?	0	1	2	3	4	5
5. ...had a weak urinary stream?	0	1	2	3	4	5
6. ...had to push or strain to begin urination?	0	1	2	3	4	5
	None	Once	Twice	3 times	4 times	5 times or more
7. Over the past month, how many times did you most typically get up to urinate from the time you went to bed at night until the time you got up in the morning?	0	1	2	3	4	5

Supplementary question – Quality of life due to urinary symptoms
If you were to spend the rest of your life with your urinary condition the way it is now, how would you feel about that?

0. Delighted
1. Pleased
2. Mostly satisfied
3. Mixed – about equally satisfied and dissatisfied
4. Mostly dissatisfied
5. Unhappy
6. Terrible

Investigations in primary care

Tests in the primary care setting should include dipstix urinalysis +/– formal culture of a midstream urine specimen (MSU), to exclude urosepsis and dipstix positive and/or microscopic haematuria, blood tests examining renal function (any evidence of obstructive renal failure should lead to immediate secondary care referral) and after the necessary informative counselling, a PSA measurement may be offered.

Further investigations (usually requested in secondary care)

Although considered optional by most urological organisations around the world, some kind of urodynamic assessment is useful as well as an estimation of efficiency of bladder emptying by ultrasonic measurement of a post-void residual volume urine volume (PVR) in a man presenting with bothersome LUTS. A urodynamic evaluation is likely to be simple and non-invasive in the first instance, in the form of uroflowmetry tests. Assuming sufficient volume of urine is passed (>125–150 ml), these uroflow tests provide the clinician with values for average flow rate and maximum flow rate (ml/s) and perhaps some idea as to diagnosis based upon the shape of the curve (a urethral stricture flow graph has a characteristic 'plateau' appearance). It is important to note, however, that there is significant test–retest variation in these non-invasive tests. Not only are patients, not surprisingly, ill at ease initially and thus see better test results with repeated testing, but also in the setting of these tests they are often asked to drink large volumes of fluid over a short period of time, resulting in an abnormal diuresis. They often have to wait their turn to void, leading to 'overfilling' of the bladder. Unsurprisingly, this situation can lead to inefficiency in bladder muscle contraction and therefore an underestimate of maximum flow rate and overestimate of post-void residual volume.

Formal ultrasound scanning of the urinary tract or indeed of the prostate via the transrectal approach are not part of any recognised guidelines; indeed some organisations actively make a point of *not* recommending these investigations. Indications for such imaging, however, may include haematuria, urosepsis, renal failure, history of urinary tract stone disease and previous surgery. The same can be said of cysto-urethroscopy, be it under local or general anaesthesia.

Management and discussion

What information have we gathered in this patient?

The 63-year-old man has an IPSS of 19 (severely symptomatic), a Quality of Life Score of 4 (dissatisfied), a PSA of 2.9 ng/ml, normal renal function (eGFR > 60), a maximum flow rate of 11 ml/s with good bladder emptying (i.e. post-void residual urine volume < 100 ml). His prostate feels enlarged and benign on DRE. He appears to drink a good volume in a 24 hour period, without evidence of nocturnal polyuria; however, his drink of choice throughout the day is tea and he likes to have a glass or two of wine in the evening.

Probably the most important information acquired during this initial evaluation of the patient relates to the exclusion of likely associated malignancy (PSA in the normal age-specific range and no evidence of haematuria) and a more accurate picture of the 'fluid habits' of the patient both in terms of what and how much is drunk and how often and what volume is voided. Evidence of excessive consumption of tea, coffee, fizzy drinks and alcohol is important, as is the total volume of fluid voided and imbibed in a 24 hour period, as (excess) consumption of such beverages can have a significant and easily reversed detrimental effect upon LUTS. Greater than 20% (younger) or 33% (the elderly) of a 'normal' 24 hour total voided volume passed at night raises the possibility of background nocturnal polyuria. The IPSS and associated quality of life score also provide an idea of how severe the patient's symptoms are and how much bother they inflict on that patient (Table 9.1). Using the IPSS the patient can be placed into mild, moderate or severe symptomatic categories. In truth, it is likely that it is this information (i.e. IPSS and quality of life score) that will have greatest influence upon management choice.

The non-invasive uroflow tests and ultrasonic estimation of post-void residual volume (PVR) will provide information regarding the likelihood of an underlying diagnosis of bladder outlet obstruction (BOO). In most age groups, a maximum flow rate of < 10 ml/s (preferably on repeat testing) has a high likelihood of confirming this diagnosis. As this figure rises, the diagnosis becomes less likely. A PVR volume in excess of 150 ml is often considered abnormal; however, as suggested above, this is a reasonably unreliable tool because of significant test–retest variation and the effects of over filling at uroflowmetry tests. Nevertheless, persistent large post-void residual volumes (e.g. in excess of 300 ml) are worrying in terms of potential detrusor (bladder muscle) failure with or without a background of BOO secondary to benign prostatic enlargement/hyperplasia (BPE/BPH).

Therefore the patient has a likely diagnosis of BOO secondary to BPE – beyond his current plight, what might it mean for him in the future?

The chance of such a patient suffering deterioration in his symptoms in the short to medium term (four years or so), or (even worse) suffering the generally unrecognised trauma associated with developing acute retention of urine, is actually quite small, roughly 7%. However, it is likely that his symptoms will deteriorate over a longer period. The chances of urinary retention are greater in those of greater age, with larger prostates, higher PSA readings, poorer flow rates and larger post-void residual volumes.

What are the treatment options for symptomatic BOO secondary to BPE?

The aim of any treatment is the relief of the patient's symptoms and improvement in quality of life, with the added potential of altering the disease progression. Naturally, most treatments are focused on the first two objectives.

Conservative management/watchful waiting

Men with a low IPSS (< 7) and little bother from their water works may want to adopt a more expectant approach in their management. However, we know that a simple approach of education and advice (particularly regarding fluid management – i.e. examining and altering what is drunk and when) can have a significant beneficial effect upon mild to moderate LUTS as defined by the IPSS. Such intervention should be considered essential in the management of all patients with LUTS and in this setting can be as effective as medical therapy. Alteration of medication with significant urinary side effects and treatment of constipation may also be helpful and is certainly of importance.

Medical therapy

In men with moderate to severe symptoms (IPSS ≥ 8) with associated bother, most guidelines suggest they should be offered either medical or surgical intervention.

The mainstays of medical therapy are the alpha-blockers and the 5-alpha reductase inhibitors:

■ alpha-blocker therapy is based upon the hypothesis that LUTS are (partially) caused by alpha 1 adrenergic mediated contraction of prostatic smooth muscle and bladder neck. Many generic options are available, becoming more and more selective for the alpha 1a receptor as newer generations were released, thus decreasing, particularly, cardiovascular side effects, namely dizziness. alpha-blockers generally lead to a 4–6 point improvement in the IPSS and a 2–2.5 ml/s improvement in maximum flow rate (approx. 25% on average). It is interesting that a surprisingly significant improvement in storage LUTS may be seen. This may be explained by the concurrent antagonism of alpha 1d receptors that are seen in the overactive detrusor in this setting. Other side effects include tiredness, asthenia, ejaculatory problems and nasal congestion.

- Finasteride and dutasteride are the currently available 5-alpha reductase inhibitors. These drugs both prevent the conversion of testosterone to its more biologically active metabolite, dihydrotestosterone (DHT) leading to definite and sustained shrinkage of the prostate gland (by on average 20%), improvement in LUTS and reduction in risk of urinary retention, need for surgery and symptom deterioration in the medium term (4–5 years). These benefits are not maintained in a similar time frame by alpha-blocker therapy. Reported side effects include loss of libido, gynaecomastia, ejaculatory dysfunction and erectile dysfunction and depending on whether finasteride (Type II antagonist) or dutasteride (Type I and II antagonist) is prescribed there may be a 6 or 3 month delay in achieving maximum benefit, respectively. Maximum benefit for either of these drugs is seen in prostate glands with a volume greater than 25–30 ml – for practical purposes that means almost all glands that feel enlarged on DRE. In fact, for those glands of such a volume (or with a PSA > 1.4) the combination of an alpha-blocker and a 5-alpha reductase inhibitor, has been shown, in a very well-designed study, to actually offer the most benefit in terms of both symptom improvement and risk reduction of those adverse events, including acute urinary retention. In truth, whilst these reductions in risk may be described as in excess of 50%, this is actually reducing the risk from roughly 7% to 3% over a five-year period for urinary retention. Furthermore, it is to be noted that a combination of these two drug families not only also means a combination of risk of side effects but also of cost and therefore financial burden.

Surgical treatment

All published guidelines suggest surgical intervention in those men with complicated LUTS, e.g. refractory urinary retention (failed at least one trial without catheter), renal failure secondary to high-pressure chronic retention, recurrent episodes of urosepsis and bladder stones due to BOO. Other candidates have traditionally also included those who refuse, have no benefit from or fail to tolerate medical therapy.

Transurethral resection of the prostate (TURP) remains in many minds the 'gold standard' option for all bar the very large prostate glands (> 80–100 ml). However, the 60–70% improvement in IPSS and the > 100% gain in maximum flow rate are matched by some of the newer, less invasive modalities available; specifically the GreenLight HPS 532 nm laser, which vaporises tissue away and the Holmium:YAG laser which is used to incise and enucleate the adenoma within the prostate, this tissue then being retrieved from the bladder after morcellation. Both these modalities can be used to treat all sizes of prostates with virtually no extra risk (unlike TURP) thanks to the minimal bleeding associated with each laser modality and the use of safer irrigant fluid. That is, a zero risk of blood transfusion or TUR syndrome, a rare but potentially fatal complication of TURP. Indeed, the haemostasis achieved with the GreenLight HPS laser system is so effective that the procedure can reliably be performed on a day case basis. This also allows, of course, a very rapid removal of any post-operative catheter (< 24 hours) and return to normal activity (after two weeks). Furthermore, both these laser modalities appear to be associated with a lower risk of side effects on sexual function, although long-term retrograde ejaculation remains likely and should really, therefore, be expected by the patient.

In the past, therefore, patients with moderate to severe symptoms who were offered a choice between medical therapy and surgical intervention almost always shied away from the clearer much greater benefits associated with a TURP/open prostatectomy in terms of symptom improvement thanks to the perceived associated morbidity of a prolonged hospital stay and catheterisation for 48–72 hours (or more!), the small risk of blood transfusion and deterioration in sexual function. The emergence of newer technologies, such as the lasers above, has meant that the surgical option has become less of a leap of faith and in the authors' experience many men are now happy to trade off the likelihood of retrograde ejaculation against the much greater improvement in LUTS and flow rate seen after these treatments and opt for surgical treatment in the first instance, because the perceived associated morbidty of that procedure has shifted to a much more acceptable place.

Key points

- A thorough medical history is very important and can be supplemented by the use of a validated questionnaire such as the International Prostate Symptom Score (IPSS), which includes a quality of life score.

- Tests in the primary care setting should include dipstix urinalysis as well as a formal culture of a midstream urine specimen. Blood tests examining renal function and, after the necessary informative counselling, a PSA measurement may be offered. A uroflow test with a post-void residual urine volume is also helpful, but is certainly not mandatory in the first instance.
- In men with mild symptoms a watchful waiting policy is often sufficient with simple advice on controlling fluid intake and avoidance of caffeinated drinks.
- In men with moderate to severe symptoms the mainstays of medical therapy are the alpha-blockers and the 5-alpha reductase inhibitors.
- In men with moderate to severe symptoms and poor quality of life score or those with complicated BPH (i.e. failure of medical therapy, resulting renal failure, bladder stones etc.) surgical intervention is advocated.
- Transurethral resection of the prostate (TURP) remains in many minds the 'gold standard' surgical option but laser prostatectomy (particularly the GreenLight laser) is fast gaining in popularity.

Further reading and bibliography

Arrighi, H. M., Metter, E. J., Guess, H. A. and Fozzard, J. L. (1991) Natural history of benign prostatic hyperplasia and risk of prostatectomy. The Baltimore Longitudinal Study of Aging. *Urology*, **38**(1 suppl.), 4–8.

Brown, C. T., Yap, T., Cromwell, D. A., Rixon, L., Steed, L., Mulligan, K., Mundy, A., Newman, S. P., van der Meulen, J. and Emberton, M. (2007) Self management for men with lower urinary tract symptoms: randomised controlled trial. *Br. Med. J.*, **334**, 25.

European Association of Urology Guidelines (2008) http://www.uroweb.org/professional-resources/guidelines/; accessed June 2008.

McConnell, J. D., Roehrborn, C. G., Bautista, O. M., Andriole, G. L. Jr, Dixon, C. M., Kusek, J. W. *et al.* (2003) Medical Therapy of Prostatic Symptoms (MTOPS) Research Group. The long-term effect of doxazosin, finasteride, and combination therapy on the clinical progression of benign postatic hyperplasia. *N. Engl. J. Med.*, **349**, 2387–98.

CHAPTER 10

Haematuria

Aza Mohammed, Blanca Martin-Retortillo, Jay Khastgir,
Sandy Gujral and Ignacio Zamora

Case history

An otherwise healthy 68-year-old male presented to his GP surgery stating that he had seen blood in his urine. The episode was painless and not associated with any urinary symptoms. The past medical history of this patient revealed hypertension for which he is on treatment and his past surgical history revealed inguinal hernia repair. The patient is not on aspirin or other antiplatelet drugs. Socially the patient is a smoker of 20 cigarettes a day for the last 40 years and he drinks alcohol in moderation. He used to work as a school teacher. On clinical examination, the patient looked healthy, with some nicotine staining of his lips and index finger. Abdominal examination was unremarkable and digital rectal examination revealed a moderately enlarged benign prostate. The patient was asked to give a urine sample which was pink in colour and strongly positive for blood on dipstix. How would you evaluate?

Introduction

Prevalence

Haematuria is defined as the presence of blood in the urine. This blood can originate from any site along the urinary tract. It could be a sign of serious underlying disease and it therefore warrants full evaluation. The prevalence of haematuria on dipstix testing in the adult population is estimated to be 2–16%.

In a large UK-based study (Khadra *et al.*, 2000; see further reading), approximately 35% of patients evaluated for macroscopic haematuria were found to have significant underlying pathology, with the incidence of cancer being 25% in these patients, whereas approximately 20% of patients with microscopic haematuria had significant pathology, of which 9.4% had neoplastic disease. Thus, due to the comparatively high percentage of patients with macroscopic haematuria who have neoplasms, we recommend that this group is referred directly to a urologist, whereas microscopic/urine dipstix positive haematuria can be initially managed in the community.

Classification and aetiology

Haematuria is broadly classified into glomerular (i.e. renal parenchymal disease) and non-glomerular (urological) causes. In this chapter we are going to discuss the non-glomerular causes of haematuria.

Haematuria can also be categorised into:

- Macroscopic: visible as frank blood, smoky or tea-coloured urine.
- Microscopic: defined as the presence of three or more red blood cells (RBCs) per high-power field on microscopic examination of urinary sediment from *two of three* properly collected urinalysis specimens. Microscopic haematuria can also be diagnosed with urine dipstix which is commonly performed in community health centres – once again at least two of three urine specimens must be dipstix positive.

The most common causes of haematuria include:

- *Kidney*: trauma, tumours (renal cell carcinoma and transitional cell carcinoma of the renal pelvis), stones, infection and cystic disease (adult polycystic kidney disease and medullary sponge kidney)
- *Ureters*: stones, infections or tumours
- *Bladder*: stones, infections or tumours
- *Prostate*: benign prostatic enlargement or prostatic cancer
- *Urethra*: stones, infections and tumours
- Other causes include:
  - Glomerular disease (acute glomerulonephritis, benign essential haematuria, benign familial haematuria, Goodpasteur's disease and amyloidosis)
  - Endometriosis
  - Strenuous exercise
  - Coagulopathy (congenital or acquired)

- Drugs (such as cyclophosphamide, non-steroidal anti-inflammatory analgesics and anticoagulant overdose)
- Metabolic disorders (hypercalciuria and hyperuricosuria)
- Renal infarction
- Renal papillary necrosis
- False haematuria (such as menstrual bleeding, food pigments or drug metabolites)

Evaluation of patients with haematuria

The aim of initial evaluation is to confirm the presence of haematuria, identify common causes and select patients with significant urinary tract pathology for further assessment (Table 10.1).

Table 10.1 The basic evaluation of patients with haematuria.

1.	History
2.	Physical examination
3.	Investigations

- Urinalysis
- Blood tests (FBC, U&Es, clotting screen)
- Urine cytology
- Urinary tract imaging (Intravenous pyelography, ultrasound, CT scan)
- Cystoscopy (flexible or rigid)

History

Valuable information could be gained by taking an accurate history from the patient. The timing of bleeding could give an idea about the origin of the bleeding – initial haematuria (at the beginning of micturition) is usually urethral in origin whilst total haematuria (throughout micturition) is usually caused by lesions arising above the bladder neck. Terminal haematuria (at the end of micturition), on the other hand, usually arises from the bladder neck or prostate as the bladder neck contracts trying to squeeze out the last amounts of urine. The presence of clots is an indication of the severity of haematuria.

The presence of pain on micturition, i.e. dysuria, is usually an indication of an inflammatory/infective process and it is less alarming than a painless haematuria, which is usually a feature of malignancy. A colicky pain in the flank radiating to the groin or the genitalia is associated with ureteric stones or the passage of clots along the ureters from an upper tract lesion. *Loin pain/ haematuria syndrome* is an idiopathic condition characterised by the presence of repeated episodes of loin pain and haematuria of varying degrees with no underlying cause. A deep-seated pelvic pain associated with marked irritative bladder symptoms is a feature of prostatic inflammation.

Patients with urinary tract malignancies and renal tuberculosis may present with generalised ill health associated with loss of appetite, loss of weight, fever and night sweating. A history of joint pains, skin rashes and prolonged fever, especially in adolescent patients, suggests a collagen vascular disorder.

The past medical and surgical histories of the patient, such as previous episodes of haematuria, genitourinary infections, urinary stones treatment, tumours, pelvic irradiation and prostatic enlargement in males should be taken into account. The presence of chronic atrial fibrillation or a recent history of myocardial infarction may indicate renal emboli and infarction. Family history could be of value as certain diseases such as polycystic disease of the kidneys, Fabry's disease, Alport's syndrome, benign essential haematuria (Berger's disease), von Hippel-Lindau disease and sickle cell trait could present as haematuria. Benign familial haematuria is an autosomal dominant condition characterised by the presence of microscopic haematuria among members of the same family. It can affect any age group (usually above the age of 32 years) and it has a two-to-one female predominance. It is associated with minimal proteinuria and has no long-term implication on renal function.

A comprehensive drug history should be taken from the patient. Many drugs can cause haematuria as a side effect such as nonsteroidal analgesics (causing papillary necrosis) and cyclophosphamide (causing haemorrhagic cystitis). Other drugs, such as rifampicin, can cause red urine, which can be mistaken for haematuria.

A history of sexually transmitted diseases, endometriosis, sexual activity, pregnancies and menstrual period should be noted. Strenuous exercise such as marathon running, swimming and other group sports can also lead to haematuria. Finally, history of smoking and occupational exposure to certain chemicals (benzidine and naphthylamine) should be noted as they increase the risk of bladder cancers.

Examination

Generally the patient should be noted for the presence of weight loss, lymphadenopathy, rashes, ecchymoses or other cutaneous lesions such as angiomas or telengectasias.

The blood pressure should be assessed for hypertension, which could indicate an underlying renal parenchymal disease. Examination of the heart for rate, rhythm or murmurs could indicate an underlying throboembolic process as a cause of haematuria. The lungs should be examined for signs of heart failure. The presence of peripheral oedema is a sign of glomerular cause of haematuria.

The abdomen should be inspected for any swelling, visible pulsations, stomas, scars of previous surgical operations, or signs of previous pelvic irradiation. Palpation of the abdomen may reveal tenderness in inflammatory conditions such as pyelonephritis or masses such as enlarged kidneys or renal masses, liver or spleen. The bladder should be percussed for dullness, which is an indication for chronic urinary retention secondary to bladder outflow obstruction. Finally careful auscultation of the abdomen may reveal bruits as result of renal artery stenosis or aneurysms. Digital rectal examination must always be performed to assess the prostate for size, consistency, contour, tenderness and the presence of nodules.

Investigations

These aim to confirm the presence of haematuria and identify any underlying cause.

Urinalysis

This is an array of tests performed on the urinary sediment and it is the initial test for patients with haematuria. The number of RBCs per high-power field should be determined. In addition the sample should be examined for the presence of dysmorphic RBCs or the presence of red cell casts which are signs of glomerular disease. As a general rule, the presence of more than 80% normal red cells is an indication of lower urinary tract bleeding while the presence of more than 80% dysmorphic red cells is an indication of a glomerular disease. Accurate determination of RBC morphology may require inverted phase contrast microscopy. This is an optical microscopy illumination technique in which small phase shifts in the light passing through a transparent specimen are converted into amplitude or contrast changes in the image. A phase contrast microscope does not require staining to view the slide. The urine sample should also be tested for the presence of proteinuria. Proteinuria is defined as a total protein excretion of more than 1 g per day or more than 500 mg per day if it is persistent or increasing or if other factors suggest the presence of renal parenchymal disease. Urine should also be tested for the presence of urinary tract infections (UTIs). This is defined as the presence of more than five white cells per high-power field or the finding at culture of more than 100,000 colonies/ml of a single organism. Those patients should be treated with antibiotics and further investigations should be deferred for six weeks. If further urinalysis reveals no haematuria then the patient would need no further evaluation.

Assessment of urea and electrolytes (U&Es)

This is useful in detecting obstruction of the urinary tract, but abnormal results may also suggest an underlying glomerular disease as a cause for haematuria.

Clotting screen

This should be performed when there is suspicion of an underlying clotting abnormality. This includes a full blood count (FBC) to detect any low platelet count. It also includes assessment of the international randomised ratio (INR) which is particularly important in patients with warfarin overdose, who may present as haematuria.

Urine cytology

Loss of cell-to-cell adhesiveness is one of the characteristics of malignant cells. This would result in constant shedding of cells from the tumour surface which can be detected in the urine. Urine cytology has low sensitivity for detecting low-grade bladder tumours, but the sensitivity for higher grade tumours and carcinoma *in situ* is markedly improved. The specificity, however, could be as high as 100% for bladder tumour detection. False-positive results are seen in patients with chronic infection, stones or recent intravesical chemotherapy or pelvic irradiation. The results can be difficult to interpret in the presence of gross haematuria. The presence of atypical or malignant cells in the urine with negative cystoscopy should alert the clinician to the presence of upper tract malignancies and further evaluation with ureteroscopy and possibly brush cytology is needed.

Urinary markers

Several urinary markers are available for detecting new or recurrent bladder cancer, e.g. nuclear matrix protein 22 (NMP-22) and bladder tumour antigen (BTA). Few of them, however, have gained FDA approval for clinical use and the available data is currently insufficient to recommend the routine use of these markers in evaluating patients with haematuria.

Urinary tract imaging

This is an essential part of the initial assessment of patients with haematuria. They are mainly used to detect kidney tumours (both renal cell carcinoma and transitional cell carcinoma of the renal pelvis), renal stones and the presence of renal infections.

These modalities include:

- **Ultrasonography (USS) plus plain X-ray**: ultrasound of the renal tract can be used as an initial screening test for patients with haematuria. It can differentiate between solid and cystic renal masses and it is very useful for the characterisation of renal cysts. It can also detect large bladder tumours and hydronephrosis. It is cheap, widely available and does not involve exposure to radiation. USS, however, is of limited use in detecting small solid lesions (less than 3 cm) and it is largely operator-dependent.

  USS is usually combined with a plain X-ray of the kidneys, ureters and bladder (KUB), which helps show up urinary tract stones.
- **Intravenous urography (IVU)**: it is considered to be the best initial study for the evaluation of the urinary tract. It is cost-effective and available in the majority of centres. It can detect renal stones and transitional cell tumour of the renal pelvis. It has a limited sensitivity for detecting small renal masses and it cannot differentiate solid and cystic lesions. It is also contraindicated in patients with contrast allergy or those with impaired renal function.
- **Computerised tomography scan (CT) with contrast**: this has largely replaced all the other modalities as an initial screening test for haematuria. It is the modality of choice for urinary stones when used without injection of contrast, with a sensitivity of 94–98%, compared to IVU which has a sensitivity of 52–59%. It is also the preferred modality for the detection and characterisation of solid renal masses (tri-phasic CT with contrast). A

CT urogram is superior to IVU in the evaluation of patients with suspected transitional cell carcinoma of the renal pelvis. In addition it is the best modality for detecting renal and peri-renal infections, e.g. renal or peri-renal abscesses. The current recommendation for the use of CT scan in the initial assessment of haematuria is to start with a non-contrast study. If the study demonstrates urolithiasis and the patient is low risk for underlying malignancy (age less than 40 years, negative urine cytology and the absence of irritative bladder symptoms), then no further scanning is required. If the patient is at high risk of developing malignancy and there is no evidence of renal stones, then CT urogram should be performed for further evaluation of the urinary tract.

- **Magnetic resonance imaging (MRI)**: rarely used in the evaluation of haematuria and considered as a problem-solving approach for patients who require additional imaging after CT or USS. MRI is more expensive and less widely available than the other modalities.

Flexible or rigid cystoscopy

This is defined as the visual evaluation of the lower urinary tract, including the urethra, ureteric orifices and the bladder mucosa. It is regarded as the gold standard for detecting bladder tumours. Initial cystoscopic study should be performed using flexible instruments as this is a simple procedure with only 2% lignocaine jelly pushed into the urethra necessary for adequate anaesthesia. It is associated with fewer complications, such as pain and injury to the lower urinary tract. In addition, positioning and preparation of the patient are much simplified, with a shorter procedure time. Flexible cystoscopy is considered ideal for an office urology setting and may be performed by an appropriately trained GP with a specialist interest (GPSI) or even a specialist nurse. Rigid instruments, however, require general anaesthesia, but allow for resection of tumours or suspicious lesions. They also allow performing additional procedures such as retrograde imaging of the upper tracts. Cystoscopy is associated with urinary tract infections in up to 5% of cases.

Management

Patients presenting to the GP with frank haematuria should be referred directly to the hospital, as up to 25% of them will have malignancy. In the hospital setting they may need a large (at least 22F) three-way urethral catheter inserted with bladder washout or irrigation to prevent the development of blood clots.

Subsequent management of haematuria is tailored to the underlying cause. It varies greatly from simple antibiotics to treat severe urinary tract infections to more radical surgery such as radical nephrectomy or nephroureterectomy for renal cell carcinoma or transitional cell carcinoma of the renal pelvis respectively or transurethral resection of bladder tumour (TURBT) and perhaps radical cystectomy for muscle invasive bladder cancers.

Patients with microscopic/urine dipstix positive haematuria can be managed initially in the community. Up to 10% may have an underlying malignancy. The GP should send MSU for culture, urine for cytology and we recommend ideally both USS of the renal tract and an IVU, as it is suggested that a significant number of malignancies may be missed if only USS or IVU alone is performed. The gold standard radiological investigation would be a CT urogram but this is not readily available at all hospitals and in most areas would need to be recommended by a urologist. The patient should also have a flexible cystoscopy either in the community by a GPSI or in the hospital setting.

In patients who have no cause for microscopic haematuria identified following initial assessment, data regarding follow-up is inadequate and recommendations regarding appropriate follow-up must be based on consensus opinion, in addition to review of the available literature-based evidence. The risk of life-threatening lesions is this group is low. We recommend that with a negative initial evaluation of asymptomatic microscopic haematuria, consideration should be given to repeating urinalysis, voided urine cytology and blood pressure determination at 6, 12, 24 and 36 months. Additional evaluation, including repeat imaging and cystoscopy, may be warranted in patients with persistent microscopic haematuria in whom there is a high index of suspicion for significant underlying disease, e.g. long-term smokers, mainly irritative voiding symptoms (can be a presenting feature of *in situ* bladder cancer), elderly patients, change to macroscopic haematuria, and previous exposure to chemicals. Otherwise the patient can be discharged after 36 months follow-up.

Any patient with micoscopic haematuria in whom urological investigations are negative and who is found to have any of the criteria listed below should have a nephrological referral for evaluation of renal parenchymal disease:

- Hypertension
- Proteinuria
- Urinary red cell casts or dysmorphic RBCs (evidence of glomerular bleeding)
- Impaired renal function

Renal biopsy is usually needed to determine the underlying pathology in these cases.

Key points

- Haematuria, either macroscopic or microscopic, is abnormal and should always be investigated.
- Approximately 25% of patients with macroscopic haematuria and 10% with microscopic haematuria will have an underlying urological malignancy.
- Macroscopic haematuria should be referred directly to the urologist, whereas microscopic haematuria can initially be investigated and managed in the community by the GP.
- The underlying cause of haematuria can often be elicited from the patient's history.
- MSU for culture, urine cytology, imaging of the upper urinary tract (USS plus IVU) and flexible cystoscopy are the essential investigations performed.
- Any patient with microscopic haematuria in whom urological investigations are negative and who is found to have either hypertension, proteinuria, urinary red cell casts or dysmorphic RBCs (evidence of glomerular bleeding) or impaired renal function should have prompt nephrological referral for evaluation of renal parenchymal disease.

Further reading and bibliography

Fickenscher, L. (1999) Evaluating adult hematuria. *Nurse Pract.*, **24**, 58–65.

Grossfeld, G. D., Litwin, M. S., Wolf, J. S. Jr *et al.* (2001) Evaluation of asymptomatic microscopic hematuria in adults: the American Urological Association best practice policy – part II: patient evaluation, cytology, voided markers, imaging, cystoscopy, nephrology evaluation, and follow-up. *Urology*, **57**, 604–10.

Khadra, M. H., Pickard, R. S., Charlton, M., Powell, P. H. and Neal, D. E. (2000) A prospective analysis of 1,930 patients with haematuria to evaluate current diagnostic practice. *J. Urol.*, **163**, 524–7.

Mariani, A. J., Mariani, M. C., Macchioni, C., Stams, U. K., Hariharan, A. and Moriera, A. (1989) The significance of adult hematuria: 1,000 hematuria evaluations including a risk-benefit and cost-effectiveness analysis. *J. Urol.*, **141**, 350–5.

NICE Clinical Guideline CG27 (2008) Referral for suspected cancer. http://www.nice.org.uk/nicemedia/pdf/CG027publicinfo.pdf; accessed June 2008.

CHAPTER 11

Bladder cancer

Andrew Robinson, Azhar Khan, Iqbal Shergill, Ann McDougall and Brian Waymont

Case history

A 60-year-old man presents to his GP with a single episode of painless gross haematuria. There is no history of associated lower urinary tract symptoms (LUTS). He was previously fit and well and on no regular medication. He smokes up to 20 cigarettes a day. Abdominal examination is normal and urine test rules out infection. Routine blood tests including full blood count, urea, creatinine and electrolytes are also normal. The patient is referred to a urologist as an urgent two-week referral and an outpatient flexible cystoscopy confirms a papillary lesion in the bladder.

Introduction

Bladder cancer is the second most common urological malignancy in the UK. The annual incidence is steadily increasing and is currently $\approx 10,000$ cases per annum. It is the fourth most common cancer in males and the eleventh most common cancer in females. Five-year relative survival rates have risen over the past 40 years in the UK, primarily due to increased awareness and early diagnosis. At the time of diagnosis most bladder cancers are localised to the bladder, but up to 15% will have nodal disease or distant metastasis.

Types of bladder cancer

The commonest bladder cancer, and the focus of this chapter, is transitional cell carcinoma (TCC). TCC accounts for > 90%. Macroscopically, in appearance, it may be papillary in nature or sessile and ulcerated. Other, rarer, types of bladder cancer are adenocarcinoma and squamous cell cancer (SCC). Less than 2% of bladder tumours are adenocarcinomas and appear solid or ulcerative macroscopically. These tend to be on the floor of the bladder and one-third are found in the urachus at the dome. These tumours are also quite aggressive and usually muscle invasive. They carry a poorer prognosis. In the UK, 1% of bladder cancer can be attributable to squamous cell carcinoma. They are usually solid, nodular or ulcerative on inspection and muscle invasive. Squamous cell carcinoma is associated with schistosomiasis, which is endemic in Africa and the Middle East, accounting for 60–70% of bladder cancer.

Who is at risk?

Bladder cancer is more common in males than females, with an incidence ratio of 3:1. Although bladder cancer has been seen in children and young adults, this is rare. The incidence increases with age and the average age at diagnosis is 65 years old. It is more commonly seen in the white population but carries a poorer prognosis in afro-caribbeans.

The main risk factors known to increase the risk of developing bladder cancer include: smoking, occupational exposure to certain chemicals, and inflammation/infection.

- **Smoking**: this is the most closely linked risk factor for developing bladder cancer in Western countries. It is believed that almost 50% of bladder cancers are caused by smoking and the risk of developing cancer is at least twice as likely in smokers as opposed to non-smokers. The carcinogens in cigarette smoke are excreted into the urine with alpha and beta-naphthylamine identified as two of the main causative agents.
- **Occupational exposure**: occupational exposure to certain chemicals and carcinogens accounts for 15–35% of cases in men and 1–6% in women. Those who have been exposed to aromatic amines in the rubber, textile, dye, leather, printing, solvent and petroleum industries are at a higher risk. It can take approximately 25 years after the exposure to certain chemicals before a bladder cancer is likely to develop. It is important that GPs are aware of this association as the patient could be entitled to claim Industrial Disease Benefit from the Department of Social Security.

■ **Inflammation/infection**: these factors are commonly associated with SCC. The presences of an indwelling catheter, bladder stones or chronic infection have all been associated with a higher risk of developing SCC. *Schistosoma haematobium* is also believed to increase the risk of SCC as Bilharziasis infection is found to be closely associated with the prevalence of SCC in Egypt.

History and presenting features

Haematuria

The most common initial presentation of bladder cancer is painless, gross haematuria. More than 80% of cases present in this way. It may present as constant or intermittent episodes, although the latter is more commonly seen. It may also present as microscopic haematuria, which is usually found on routine urine dipstix testing. It is estimated that 7–13% of those over 50 years old with microscopic haematuria will be suffering from a urological malignancy. If further repeat dipstix testing does not show haematuria this does not rule out a bladder cancer because, as mentioned before, the haematuria is usually intermittent. All patients found to have haematuria should be thoroughly and urgently investigated in order to rule out or achieve an early diagnosis of a urinary tract malignancy.

Lower urinary tract symptoms (LUTS)

Less often, patients may also present with irritative lower urinary tract symptoms such as dysuria, urgency and increased frequency. These are usually found in the presence of carcinoma *in situ* (CIS) or advanced bladder cancer. These symptoms may also be caused by urinary tract infections and therefore if they do not settle with appropriate treatment, or haematuria persists afterwards, further investigations will be needed to determine the cause.

Symptoms of advanced disease

Loin pain may be a presenting complaint if a bladder tumour has caused an obstruction to a ureter and resulted in hydronephrosis. The patient may complain of lower limb swelling secondary to iliac vessel compression from a tumour or lymphatic obstruction. Bone pain may be an indication of metastatic disease.

Examination and clinical findings

Clinical examination is usually unremarkable. There may be a few identifiable signs but these would normally be associated with advanced cancer or metastatic disease. The patient may appear pale if suffering from anaemia. This may be caused by blood lost from haematuria, chronic renal failure or bone marrow infiltration secondary to metastatic disease. On examining the abdomen a mass may be felt suprapubically or also on rectal and vaginal examination. These would only be found in large advanced cancers or locally advancing carcinomas, e.g. to the prostate or cervix. It is also important to check for lymphadenopathy or hepatomegaly, although again these would only be found in metastatic disease. It is rare to find many clinical signs on examining a patient with a superficial bladder cancer.

Management and discussion

Whom to refer and when to refer?

NICE have produced guidelines for GPs to help them decide which patients need to be seen urgently by a urologist. The symptoms that NICE say need urgent specialist referral are:

1. Macroscopic haematuria (any age or sex) with no symptoms of urine infection
2. Macroscopic haematuria with other symptoms, after urine infection has been ruled out by the GP
3. Urine infection that won't go away or keeps coming back, and with blood in the urine, in anyone over 40
4. Microscopic haematuria for no apparent reason (age > 50)
5. Abdominal mass that GP thinks could be related to the urinary tract

However, as discussed in Chapter 10, we have suggested that patients falling into categories 3 and 4 above can initially be investigated by the GP in the community.

How is it diagnosed?

Urine dipstix and MSU

These simple, non-invasive tests should be the initial starting point of investigating a patient presenting with haematuria or LUTS. They may confirm the presence of a UTI and if symptoms persist after appropriate treatment with antibiotics then further investigations would be indicated.

Urine cytology

This is an inexpensive and non-invasive investigation. It is useful in diagnosing and monitoring the progress of high-grade tumours or CIS. It is not particularly accurate in detecting low-grade superficial tumours, as there is a high rate of false negative results (40–70%).

Ultrasound

This is a non-invasive form of imaging which is commonly used in first-line investigation of haematuria. It avoids exposure to intravenous contrast and is able to identify renal masses. Hydronephrosis may be detected if a tumour is causing a ureteric obstruction, and bladder filling defects, caused by large bladder tumours, may also be identified. USS is generally combined with IVU in the investigation of haematuria (otherwise a significant number of malignancies may be missed).

Intravenous urogram (IVU)

This contrast study may demonstrate filling defects in the bladder as well as in the kidneys and ureters. This investigation is discussed further in Chapters 7 and 10.

CT urogram

This is now the gold standard investigation in investigation of haematuria (particularly frank or gross haematuria) and in the diagnosis and staging of urinary tract

TCC. It avoids the need for USS and IVU. However, it is not readily available in many hospitals and involves a significant radiation exposure. It would normally have to be requested by a urologist rather than a GP for diagnostic purposes.

Flexible cystoscopy

This remains the 'gold standard' in identifying and visualising a suspected bladder tumour. It is performed under local anaesthetic in an outpatient setting either by a GP with a specialist interest or a member of the urology team. If a tumour is identified patients will subsequently be scheduled to have a rigid cystoscopy under general anaesthetic, where a biopsy or transurethral resection of bladder tumour (TURBT) can be performed.

Staging the disease

Magnetic resonance imaging (MRI) is suggested to be more accurate than *CT imaging* in assessing the extent of progression and staging of a muscle invasive carcinoma, although both are reliable. These forms of imaging may also demonstrate regional lymphadenopathy when metastatic disease is suspected. *Chest X-ray* may be used as a staging investigation to look for evidence of distant metastases. *Bone scan* is used to detect metastatic bone deposits in patients with muscle invasive carcinoma who exhibit symptoms or altered blood tests suggesting bone metastases.

Other investigations

A *full blood count* (FBC) may show low haemoglobin and deranged *urea and electrolytes* may be found in renal failure, e.g. secondary to an obstructed ureter. *Liver function tests* (LFTs), *alkaline phosphatase* and *calcium* (Ca) levels may also be useful in detecting metastatic disease in advanced carcinoma.

Treatment of bladder cancer

Bladder tumours are graded using the 1973 WHO grading system. They can be classified as G1, G2 and G3, which corresponds to well, moderately and

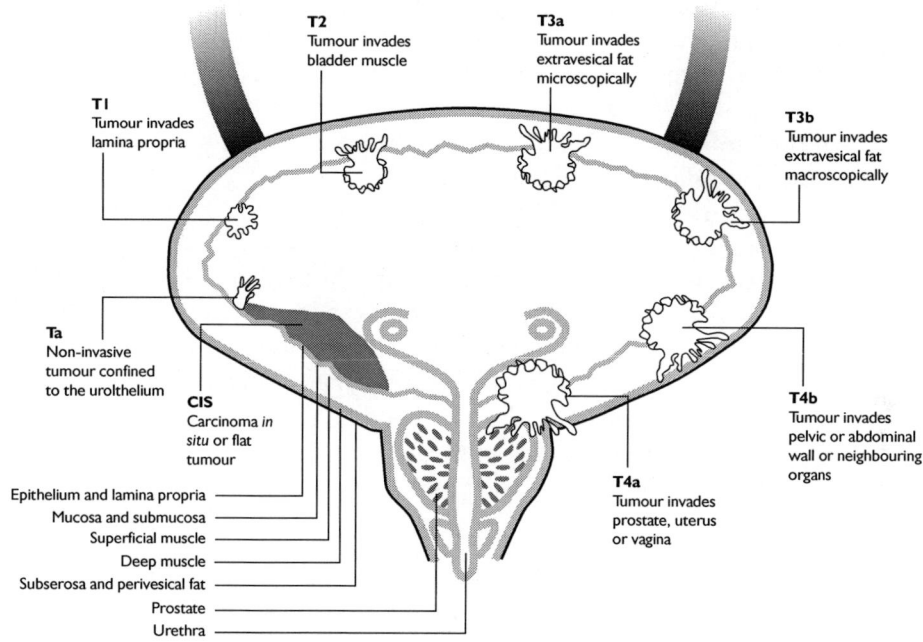

Figure 11.1 TNM staging of bladder cancer.

poorly differentiated tumour. The TNM (Tumour, Node, Metastases) staging system is widely accepted as the primary reference to the staging of a bladder cancer (Figure 11.1) and enables estimation of the prognosis and selection of appropriate treatment.

Possible discussion points with the patient

Although the GP and urologist both play an essential role in bladder cancer management, and together with other health professionals they have the freedom to clinically tailor management strategies for the specific needs of an individual patient depending on the stage of the bladder cancer, involvement of the patient in determining the most appropriate treatment strategy should be ensured. The following factors should be discussed with the patient by the healthcare professional when determining an appropriate management option:

- Smoking history and cessation advice
- Likelihood of recurrence/progression

- Life expectancy and fitness for radical treatment
- Treatment side effects
- Provide and present recommendations
- Impact on quality of life
- Patient preference
- Palliative care referral if needed
- Check for understanding and agreement

From the management point of view, bladder cancer can be broadly divided into low-grade superficial (< T2) disease, high-grade (G3) superficial disease and carcinoma *in situ* (CIS) and muscle-invasive tumours (≥ T2). Figure 11.2 summarises the primary treatments for various types of bladder cancer. These treatments are performed in secondary care although the patient may present themselves to the GP initially if there are any complications. Additionally, the GP may be involved in long-term follow-up.

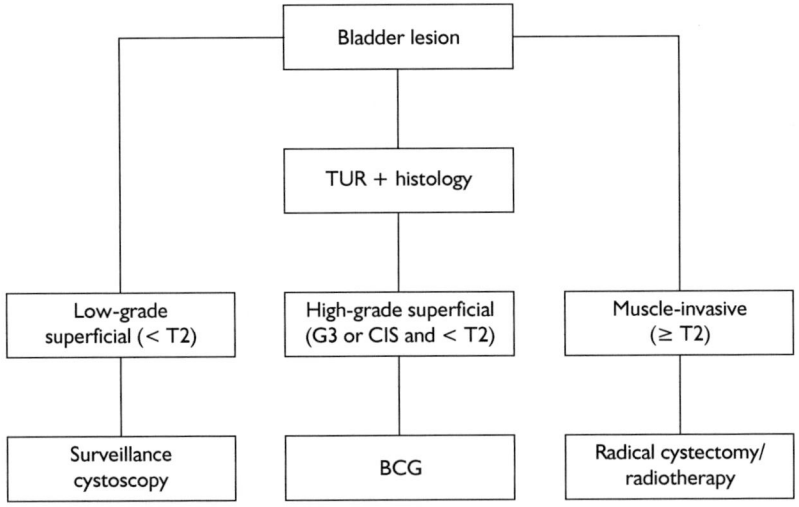

Figure 11.2 Primary management of bladder cancer.

Patient with superficial bladder cancer

The usual management for a patient with superficial disease is transurethral resection (TUR) followed by a single instillation of intravesical chemotherapy (mitomycin) to reduce the disease recurrence. This procedure is performed under general anaesthetic with a rigid cystoscope and remains the primary initial intervention in diagnosing and treating TCC of the bladder. The patient also needs to be aware that it might not be possible to remove the whole tumour. Repeat TUR may be needed and recurrence of bladder TCC is very common. Because of the high recurrence rate (60–70%), it is mandatory to perform follow-up check cystoscopies. A commonly used regimen involves cystoscopy at 3 months after initial TUR, followed by every 6 months for 2 years, and yearly thereafter throughout the patient's life.

High grade (G3) superficial disease and carcinoma *in situ* (CIS)

Intravesical BCG (Bacillus Calmette-Guerin) is the standard treatment for patients with CIS and Grade 3 superficial disease. It is an attenuated strain of *Mycobacterium bovis*; its effects are immunologically mediated and it evokes an inflammatory response within the bladder. It helps reduce the rate of reoccurrence as well as tumour progression. For patients with recurrence or no response, many urologists would perform early cystectomy to maximise survival.

Patient with muscle-invasive bladder cancer

If the histology after TUR shows high-grade T2 disease, the most commonly used treatment option is either radical cystectomy or external beam radiotherapy. Radical cystectomy involves the removal of the bladder and nearby organs. This includes the prostate gland and seminal vesicles in males, or the cervix, uterus and ovaries in females. As a radical cystectomy involves the removal of the entire bladder it is necessary to create a system for urinary diversion. These can be either continent or incontinent diversion using intestinal segment.

External beam radiation therapy has been shown to be inferior to radical cystectomy but in patients who are unsuitable candidates for surgery (age/comorbidities) it still offers a curative potential and will allow bladder preservation. The overall five-year survival rate after treatment with external beam radiation is 20–40% compared to a 90% five-year survival after cystectomy for organ-confined disease.

Management of patients with advanced/metastatic bladder cancer is primarily palliative. Radiotherapy or palliative surgery can be employed for local control, whereas short courses of radiotherapy can provide effective palliation of the symptoms of painful metastatic bone disease. Systemic chemotherapy also plays an important role in the palliative therapy of patients with multiple metastases. In addition, GPs and nurse practitioners may play an important role in providing support to patients with metastatic bladder cancer.

Key points

- Bladder cancer is the second most common urological malignancy in the UK. Improving the awareness leading to early detection is essential to improve survival.
- Smoking is the most common risk factor for developing bladder cancer in Western countries, which is thought to cause bladder cancer in 50% of men and 30% of women.
- Bladder cancer presents with painless gross haematuria in 80% of patients, but can be associated with other presentations such as microscopic haematuria, urinary symptoms and, rarely, systemic symptoms.
- Transitional cell carcinoma is the commonest form of bladder cancer, and flexible cystoscopy under local anaesthesia is the 'gold standard' to diagnose bladder cancer.
- From a management point of view, bladder cancer can be broadly divided into superficial (< T2), carcinoma *in situ* (CIS) and muscle-invasive tumours (≥ T2), but involvement of the patient in determining the most appropriate treatment strategy is essential.

Further reading and bibliography

Cancer Research UK (2008) UK Bladder Cancer Statistics. http://info.cancerresearchuk.org/cancerstats/types/bladder/; accessed June 2008.

NICE Referral Guidance for Suspected Bladder Cancer (2008) http://www.nice.org.uk/guidance/CG27/niceguidance/pdf/English; accessed June 2008.

Representatives of BAUS/BUG (2008) MDT (Multi-disciplinary Team) guidance for managing bladder cancer. British Association of Urological Surgeons (BAUS) Section of Oncology and British Uro-oncology Group (BUG). http://www.bauslibrary.co.uk/; accessed June 2008.

Masood, S., Wazait, M., Arya, M. and Patel, H. R. H. (2004) Update on bladder cancer. In *Urological Oncology: a Day-to-day Guide for the Non-Specialist* (ed. H. R. H. Patel), pp. 42–52. London: Quay Books.

CHAPTER 12

Testicular cancer

Simon Gill, Hashim Uddin Ahmed, Shashi Kumar, Manit Arya and Jayanta Barua

Case history

A 30-year-old Caucasian presents to the general practitioner with a left scrotal swelling. There is a history of trauma to the area (in hindsight, this has only drawn his attention to a painless testicular lump which might have been there for some time). There is past medical history of cryptorchism, which was surgically corrected when he was a child.

There is no history of inguinal hernia or subfertility. His father had testicular cancer.

On examination, the patient had an obvious left scrotal swelling, which one could 'get above'. The testis was not palpable separately from the mass. The swelling did not have an expansive cough impulse nor did it transilluminate.

Blood tests showed no elevations in any of the testicular tumour markers i.e. alpha-fetoprotein (AFP), beta-human chorionic gonado-trophin (β-hCG) and lactate dehydrogenase (LDH). The patient had a testicular ultrasound, which demonstrated a left intratesticular mass with a heterogenous appearance and speckled calcification. These find-ings were consistent with a testicular tumour. The patient was referred urgently to a urologist and a chest radiograph was organised, which showed no pulmonary deposits. Also, abdomino-pelvic computer tom-ography (CT) demonstrated no evidence of metastases. Thus a Stage I testicular tumour (using the Royal Marsden Staging system) was diag-nosed.

The patient consented to a radical inguinal orchidectomy. Histologi-cal analysis of the operative sample suggested a seminomatous germ cell tumour. The patient was then offered adjuvant radiotherapy to his retroperitoneum (para-aortic nodes), which he is still undergoing. This patient has a 97% five-year survival rate and has been advised to regularly perform testicular self-examination and attend outpatient follow-up.

Introduction

Testicular neoplasms account for only 1–2% of all male cancers but are the commonest tumour in 20–35 year-old men, excluding leukaemias. The incidence is approximately 1–2 cases per 100,000 population per year and prevalence is 5 cases per 100,000 population. The incidence has nearly doubled in the UK since 1971. This may be caused by endogenous or environmental oestrogenic compounds that affect the embryonic testis and increase the subsequent risk of carcinogenesis.

There are several histological types of testicular tumours (Figure 12.1), each with their own characteristics and treatments. Seminomas arise from seminiferous tubules, with metastasis spreading via lymphatics to para-aortic lymph nodes. Teratomas arise of primitive germinal cells, and thus can contain a variety of tissues, including cartilage, bone muscle and fat.

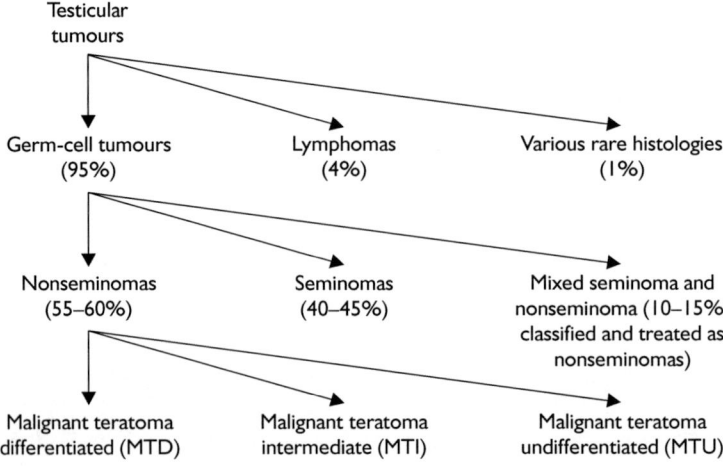

Figure 12.1 The classification of testicular cancer based on histology.

Risk factors are:

- Age: with a double peak in incidence in the young and middle-aged men. Generally, teratomas occur in the 20–30 year-old age group, seminomas occur in the 30–40 year-olds and the lymphomas in the 60–70 year-olds.
- Race: causasians have an increased risk. The American white population has approximately three times the risk of American blacks.
- Positive family history (e.g. in siblings): 6–10 times increased risk.
- History of contralateral testicular cancer: 28 times increased risk.
- Undescended testis: approximately 4 times increased risk if orchidectomy not performed. Correction of this before the age of four years is ideal, but still a higher than baseline risk remains.
- Gonadal abnormalities/dysgenesis (e.g. Klinefelter syndrome).
- Infantile hernia.
- Testicular microlithiasis – controversial.

History and examination

The differential diagnosis of a scrotal swelling is discussed in another chapter. However, it is important to point out that any painless intratesticular swelling is cancer until proved otherwise (as, similarly, an acute, tender enlargement of the testis is torsion until proved otherwise). Additionally, patients with epididymo-orchitis or orchitis who have not improved within two weeks should be referred for an urgent urological opinion according to the Clinical Oncology Information Network – this is because up to 10% of testicular tumours present in this manner.

There may be an acquired hydrocoele. There may be a history of trauma but this is likely to have drawn the patient's attention to the painless lump. Lymphatic drainage of the testis is to the para-aortic lymph nodes – this means that the inguinal lymph nodes are only enlarged when the scrotal skin is involved. Supra-clavicular lymph nodes may also be enlarged at an advanced stage.

Investigations

Serum tumour markers are important in diagnosis, prognosis and in monitoring the response to treatment. The three main tumour markers are AFP, which is produced from yolk sac cells; β-hCG expressed by trophoblasts; and LDH (isoenzyme 1), which is a marker of tumour bulk. AFP is normally found in minimal quantitities, < 100 ng/l, after the first year of life and serum levels of the beta unit of hCG should be < 5 mIU/ml. Approximately 10% of seminomas have elevated hCG levels (AFP levels are never raised in pure seminomas), whilst 90% of nonseminomatous germ cell tumours have either elevated hCG and/or AFP levels. LDH is proportional to cancer volume and is elevated in 80% of advanced cancers. Note that negative tumour marker levels do not exclude the diagnosis of a germ-cell tumour.

With regard to imaging, testicular ultrasound confirms the diagnosis in most cases. On testicular ultrasound, malignant lesions are often heterogenous and cystic, and may have speckled calcification. Chest radiograph demonstrates pulmonary deposits or mediastinal lymphadenopathy. CT scan of the chest, abdomen and pelvis provides more detailed staging information and also plays an important role in post-operative follow-up. For reference there are two staging systems for testicular tumours: the Royal Marsden Hospital Staging System and the TNM classification (Tables 12.1 and 12.2 respectively). The former is often used due to its simplicity.

Positron emission tomography is sometimes used in detecting residual masses after treatment of advanced disease.

Also, pre-treatment semen storage is often discussed and advocated.

Table 12.1 Royal Marsden Hospital Staging System for testicular tumours.

Stage	Details		
I	+/– M	Confined to testis	+/– Rising serum markers
II	A	Lymph nodes involved below the diaphragm	< 2 cm
	B		2–5 cm
	C		> 5 cm
III	A, B, C	Lymph nodes involved below and above the diaphragm	As for stage II
	M		Mediastinal
	N		Supra-clavicular, axillary or cervical
	O		No abdominal
IV	LI	Liver, lung or brain metastasis	Lung < 3 metastasis
	L2		Lung > 3 metastasis, all <2 cm
	L3		Lung > 3 metastasis, one > 2 cm
	H+		Liver
	Br+		Brain
	Bo+		Bone

Table 12.2 TNM staging system for testicular tumours.

pT	Primary tumour
pTX	Primary tumour cannot be assessed
pT0	No evidence of primary tumour (e.g. histological scar in testis)
pTis	Intratubular germ cell neoplasia (carcinoma in situ)
pT1	Tumour limited to testis/epididymis without vascular/lymphatic invasion: tumour may invade tunica albuginea but not tunica vaginalis
pT2	Tumour limited to testis/epididymis with vascular/lymphatic invasion, or tumour extending into tunica albuginea tunica vaginalis
pT3	Tumour invades spermatic cord +/– vascular/lymphatic invasion
pT4	Tumour invades scrotum +/– vascular/lymphatic invasion
N	**Regional lymph nodes clinical**
NX	Regional lymph nodes cannot be assessed
N0	No regional lymph node metastasis
N1	Metastasis with a lymph node mass ≤ 2 cm in greatest dimension or multiple lymph nodes, none > 2 cm
N2	Metastasis with a lymph node mass > 2 cm but ≤ 5 cm in greatest dimension, or multiple lymph nodes, any one mass > 2 cm but ≤ 5 cm.
N3	Metastasis with a lymph node mass > 5 cm
pN	**Pathological**
pNX	Regional lymph nodes cannot be assessed
pN0	No regional lymph node metastasis
pN1	Metastasis with a lymph node mass ≤ 2 cm and 5 or fewer positive nodes, none > 2 cm
pN2	Metastasis with a lymph node mass > 2 cm but ≤ 5 cm; or more than 5 nodes positive, ≤ 5 cm; or evidence of extranodal extension of tumour
pN3	Metastasis with a lymph node mass > 5 cm
M	**Distant metastasis**
MX	Distant metastasis cannot be assessed
M0	No distant metastasis
M1	Distant metastasis
M1a	Non-regional lymph node(s) or lung
M1b	Other sites
S	**Serum tumour markers**
Sx	Serum marker studies not available or not performed
S0	Serum marker study levels within normal limits

S	LDH (U/l)	hCG (mIU/ml)	AFP (ng/ml)
S1	$< 1.5 \times N$	and $< 5,000$	and $< 1,000$
S2	$1.5–10 \times N$	or 5,000–50,000	or 1,000–10,000
S3	$> 10 \times N$	or $> 50,000$	or $> 10,000$
	N indicates the upper limit of normal for LDH assay		

Management and discussion

Treatment is based on staging and histological type of the testicular tumour and is summarised in Table 12.3. Radical inguinal orchidectomy involves occlusion of the spermatic cord before mobilisation of the testis, thus preventing embolisation of tumour cells. Pre-procedure semen storage is often performed. It is important to note, however, that if pre-operative staging CXR or CT demonstrates large volume metastatic disease, this is classified as an oncological emergency and urgent review by an oncologist is necessary, as in these cases immediate chemotherapy may be necessary prior to surgery.

Seminomas

- Stage I: Following radical inguinal orchidectomy a surveillance protocol can be instituted in selected cases. Approximately 20% of patients overall will have micrometastases and may therefore relapse. The need for adjuvant therapy is decided by risk stratification of the tumour, e.g. tumours > 4 cm in size and those involving the rete testis are given adjuvant ipsilateral para-aortic radiotherapy (seminomas are exquisitely radiosensitive) or 1 cycle of platinum-based chemotherapy, which decreases relapse rates to 1–3%.
- Stage IIA or IIB: adjuvant radiotherapy to para-aortic and ipsilateral pelvic regions.
- Advanced disease. Three cycles of bleomycin, etoposide and cisplatin (BEP) chemotherapy. Side-effects of BEP chemotherapy reflect decreased production of bone-marrow cells. These include reduced platelets red and white cell production leading to bruising, anaemia and immunosuppression, respectively. In addition, nausea, vomiting, diarrhoea and alopecia due to reduced production of gastrointestinal and hair cells respectively may also occur.

Nonseminomatous germ cell tumours

- Stage I: 30% have subclinical metastasis, hence are at risk of relapse after radical inguinal orchidectomy. Once again, those with highest risk of relapse, i.e. presence of vascular invasion or presence of embryonal tumour, are offered adjuvant therapy in the form of 2–3 cycles of BEP or even nerve sparing retroperitoneal lymph node dissection (RPLND). This decreases relapse rates to 2–3%.

Table 12.3 A summary table of testicular tumour treatment based on type and staging of the lesion.

Histological type	Seminomatous germ cell tumours			Nonseminomatous germ cell tumours	
Royal Marsden Hospital Stage	I	IIA or IIB (metastatic)	> IIB (advanced)	I	II–IV
TNM Stage	T+	N+	M+	pT1–4	N+ and/or M+
Tumour markers	hCG			hCG or AFP	
Treatment	Radical inguinal orchidectomy plus surveillance or in high risk cases adjuvant radiotherapy to para-aortic nodes or one cycle of platinum based chemotherapy	Adjuvant radiotherapy to para-aortic and pelvic regions	Adjuvant chemotherapy – three cycles of BEP	Radical inguinal orchidectomy plus surveillance or in high risk cases adjuvant BEP (2–3 cycles) or RPLND	3–4 cycles of adjuvant BEP +/– surgical resection of residual tumour mass or initial RPLND.

■ Stages II–IV. These patients are given 3–4 cycles of adjuvant BEP or RPLND. Note that after chemotherapy surgical resection of residual para-aortic tumour mass is only indicated if that mass is greater than 1 cm and tumour markers are normalising.

Prognosis

Stage 1 seminomatous germ cell tumours have a 95% five-year survival, whilst over stage 1 this drops to 75% five-year survival. For non-seminomatous germ cell tumours stage 1, five-year survival is 90%, and in more advanced disease, survival drops to 45%.

Follow-up

Regular contralateral testicular self-examination is essential. Outpatient serial AFP, β-hCG and LDH levels with intermittent CT scanning is recommended. Note that the serum half-life of AFP and β-hCG is five to seven and two to three days respectively.

Summary

The general practitioner should have the highest suspicion for patients with painless intratesticular swellings, which should be presumed to be a neoplasm until proved otherwise. The patient should be sent for serum AFP, hCG and LDH levels and a testicular USS should be requested on an urgent basis. If the diagnosis is confirmed referral to a urologist should be immediate. The urologist would then arrange staging CT and counsel the patient for sperm banking and radical inguinal orchidectomy. It should be noted, however, that if pre-operative staging CXR or CT demonstrates large volume metastatic disease, this is an oncological emergency as immediate chemotherapy may be necessary prior to any surgery. Otherwise, adjuvant radiotherapy or chemotherapy may be necessary. Post-operative follow-up would include regular serum tumour marker levels and CTs. Importantly, the patient is taught to perform regular testicular examination of the contralateral testis.

Key points

■ In general, an acute, tender enlargement of the testis is torsion until proved otherwise.

■ Any lump within the tunica-vaginalis is cancer until proved otherwise.

■ Negative tumour marker levels do not exclude the diagnosis of a germ-cell tumour.

■ Testicular ultrasound is helpful to differentiate testicular tumours from epididymal cysts.

■ Testicular cancer should be viewed as curable.

Further reading and bibliography

Lee, F., Arya, M. and Patel, H. R. (2004). Testicular cancer: update and controversies. In: *Urological Oncology: a Day-to-day Guide For The Non-specialist* (ed. H. R. Patel), pp. 62–81. Quay Books, London.

CHAPTER 13

Prostate specific antigen (PSA)

Richard Hindley and David Love

Case history

A 58-year-old has a PSA test performed at a routine health screen and the result is elevated at 5.8 ng/ml. He has very little in the way of troublesome lower urinary tract symptoms (LUTS).

Referral to secondary care with possible prostate cancer would be appropriate for this asymptomatic man with a raised (age matched) PSA. In an asymptomatic patient, PSA should only be measured after he has been provided with all the information about the limitations of the test and the implications of an abnormal result. In this situation PSA should only be measured in men who may benefit from curative treatment of early disease; in general those with a reasonable life expectancy.

What is PSA?

PSA is a protein produced selectively by the prostate, but not specifically in prostate cancer (see Table 13.1).

The role of PSA in seminal fluid is to liquefy the semen after it has been deposited in the vagina – it enables the sperm to swim to the ova. The amount of PSA in the blood is dependent on the size of the prostate and the integrity of the 'barrier' between serum and prostate. Interestingly, a prostate cancer cell actually produces less PSA than a benign one but the integrity of the cell membrane is also important; disruption of the prostatic architecture in cancer increases the serum PSA, although prostate cancer is only one of the causes of abnormal PSA levels.

Table 13.1 Causes of an elevated PSA (other than cancer).

Factor	Comments
Benign prostatic enlargement	A larger gland will generally produce more PSA
Urinary tract infection	It is essential to exclude infection ideally before checking the PSA level
Prostatitis	Inflammation of the prostate can affect men of all ages and is not just caused by bacterial infection
Prostatic surgery and urethral instrumenta-tion	Urologists are careful to avoid PSA testing too soon after flexible cystoscopy or catheterisation
Prostate biopsy and massage	Significant manipulation of the prostate can raise PSA but **DRE alone appears to have no effect**
Ejaculation	A slight elevation occurs peaking at 1 hour after ejaculation
Cycling	This is the only form of exercise thought to influence PSA levels

In the blood PSA is inactivated by binding to proteins (complexed PSA) although some PSA circulates in an unbound form (free PSA). The standard PSA measurements detect the total of both complexed and free PSA; selective measurement of these isoforms can improve the specificity of the test and so are sometimes used by urologists to decide whether or not proceeding to biopsy is appropriate.

Defining the normal range for PSA is difficult and a cut-off level should be used that gives a reasonable yield of prostate cancer (traditionally this range was 0–4 ng/ml). An improvement on this is to provide a risk assessment for the individual that includes age, race and digital rectal examination (DRE) result. It is important also to remember that different laboratory assays from different manufacturers vary in the reference ranges they give for PSA. The incidence of prostate cancer with different ranges of PSA is shown in Table 13.2.

Table 13.2 Chance of prostate cancer on biopsies with different ranges of PSA.

	Probability of prostate cancer on biopsies				
PSA (ng/ml)	0.1–1.0	1.1–2.5	2.6–4.0	4–10	> 10
Normal DRE	1%	5%	15%	25%	> 50%
Abnormal DRE	5%	15%	30%	45%	> 75%

It is normal for the PSA level to increase with age and so whilst a PSA of 5.8 would be raised for a man in his 50s – it would be within the accepted normal range for a man in his 80s (as is discussed later in this chapter).

Screening for prostate cancer

The principle of screening for prostate cancer is to diagnose prostate cancer early with the assumption that the earlier the cancer is detected the easier it is to treat and the more likely it will be curable. From the late 1980s when serum PSA became widely available the arguments for and against screening for prostate cancer have been argued with increasing vigour. PSA has already been widely adopted in the evaluation of men presenting for health checks, but there is currently no national screening programme for prostate cancer in the UK. The fundamental question about PSA screening has always been: will it reduce mortality from prostate cancer? With recent improvements in the diagnosis and treatment of early prostate cancer perhaps the question of whether a cancer diagnosed early will lead to more appropriate management for that individual, with resulting reduced morbidity should also be asked.

Observational studies of screening

Observational screening studies have usually included PSA $\geq$ 4 ng/ml, DRE and trans-rectal ultrasound (TRUS) in men $\geq$ 50, with biopsies offered to those with an elevated PSA and/or abnormal DRE. Serum PSA was found to be $\leq$ 4 ng/ml in 88%, 4–9.9 ng/ml in 10% and > 10 ng/ml in 2% of the populations screened. The sensitivity and positive predictive value (PPV) of a PSA $\geq$ 4 ng/ml for prostate cancer are of the order of 79–82% and 32–40% respectively. This translates to approximately one-third of men with an abnormal PSA having cancer detected on systematic prostate biopsy.

The striking decline in prostate cancer mortality in the USA compared with the UK in 1994–2004 coincided with much higher uptake of the PSA test in the USA. Explanations for these different trends include the possibility of early screening of men with more aggressive asymptomatic disease in the USA. However, we should be cautious in our interpretation of mortality data from the post-PSA era. The only studies that are designed to provide direct evidence to support or refute the argument that early diagnosis significantly reduces the death rate are randomised trials of screening. Two such trials are currently in progress, the European Randomised Study of Screening for prostate Cancer (ERSPC) and the American National Cancer Institute screening project for prostate, lung, colon, and ovarian cancer (PLCO). The first results from these two large studies are reporting in the next few years. The American PCLO study has already provided useful information as to the natural history of the PSA value over time in a population of men screened annually.

The health technology assessment panel of the NHS Executive commissioned and supported two independent reviews on 'Diagnosis, management and screening of early prostate cancer' and 'The diagnosis, management, treatment and costs of prostate cancer in England and Wales'. Both reviews expressed concerns that the criteria for this screening tool had not been met, and also that the PSA test is not sufficiently accurate. There is a paucity of knowledge on prediction of tumour progression as well as the best form of treatment, in addition to the cost issues. Currently, the NHS position on PSA screening in the UK is ambiguous; whilst there is media encouragement and political support for self-determined screening, in the UK the use of PSA testing for mass screening purposes is not sanctioned.

The government has introduced a prostate cancer risk management profile for men. This aims to provide men with balanced information about the pros and cons of putting themselves forwards for a test. The Department of Health advises doctors only to use the test for checking a patient with troublesome urinary symptoms or if the patient has no symptoms but wishes to have test and is fully informed about the risks and benefits of testing. Thus it is important that *asymptomatic* patients understand and are counselled regarding the following key points prior to being offered a PSA test:

1. PSA test is not specific for prostate cancer and thus a false positive result is possible and up to three-quarters of men with a raised PSA do not have prostate cancer.
2. A false negative result is possible as the PSA test is not 100% sensitive.
3. If prostate biopsies are necessary they are associated with complications, including a 1% risk of systemic sepsis.
4. If prostate cancer is diagnosed there is uncertainty about the best way to treat it.

If PSA was used as a screening test, it is likely that some men who did not have prostate cancer would undergo unnecessary prostate biopsy. Like any invasive test, prostate biopsy can be uncomfortable and does have risks (haematuria, sepsis) and in itself is not wholly reliable; some men needing further biopsies even if the first or indeed second sets are clear of cancer. Furthermore, as greater understanding of the natural history of prostate cancer develops, so we are beginning to realise that we have probably been over treating some screen-detected prostate cancers as they were unlikely to affect the lifespan of the individual.

Enhancing the usefulness of PSA

PSA specificity

Despite the ability of PSA to detect prostate cancer, its positive predictive value is enhanced considerably when combined with DRE and so this is essential prior to referral to a urologist for all men with an elevated PSA or indeed troublesome lower urinary tract symptoms and a normal PSA. By increasing the PSA cut-off point the specificity is improved, but at the cost of decreasing sensitivity. In other words, more men without cancer will be spared further investigation, but fewer men with prostate cancer will be diagnosed. Given that approximately one quarter of men newly diagnosed with prostate cancer have a normal PSA level, attempts to improve the performance of PSA would seem sensible. Avoiding false positive PSA testing is important as this avoids unnecessary biopsy with its associated costs both psychological and financial. If the PSA level is borderline (when matched for age) then it would be reasonable to repeat the PSA prior to referral if the DRE is normal and there is otherwise no cause for concern. A PSA rise that is suspected to be due to infection does not necessitate urgent referral *per se*, but will require referral for investigation by a urologist (cystoscopy and ultrasound) with a follow-up PSA.

Age-related PSA

PSA rises with increasing age, mainly as a result of prostatic enlargement but also because the amount of 'activity' within the gland also increases, which causes leakage of PSA from the lumen of prostate. Using the PSA range for an older man will avoid unnecessary concern and intrusive investigation (Table 13.3). The main problem with age-specific ranges is that they don't take into account the rising incidence of prostate cancer with advancing age. Increasing the threshold for biopsy in the older patients will inevitably reduce the number of cancers detected; however, this is not necessarily cause for concern as with

Table 13.3 Age-related PSA levels.

Age (years)	PSA range* (ng/ml)
50–59	0–3.0
60–69	0–4.0
≥ 70	0–5.0

*The ranges may vary slightly from one clinical biochemistry laboratory to another

reducing life expectancy the likelihood of dying from missed prostate cancer decreases (14% of all men are diagnosed with prostate cancer, but only 4% of all men will die from prostate cancer).

PSA density

PSA is also helpful in assessing the size of the prostate gland (particularly in men < 70 years) in men with suspected symptomatic benign prostate enlargement. Larger glands are more likely to give rise to higher serum PSA levels. If the volume of the prostate gland is known (this is usually measured by ultrasound) the PSA density (PSAD) can be calculated. It is derived from the PSA level divided by the volume of the gland and a PSAD of ≤ 0.15 ng/ml is favourable if the PSA is in the range 4–10 ng/ml; there are conflicting reports as to the usefulness of this test with regard to when to use it and what cut-off to use. There may be a better correlation between the size of the transition zone and the likelihood of a positive biopsy in patients with a borderline PSA, given that it is the transition zone that enlarges with ageing.

If at the time of referral for biopsy the patient discussed at the start of this chapter was discovered to have a large prostate gland (of the order of 158 ml) with a normal DRE then the PSAD would be calculated with a favourable density ($5.8 \div 150 = 0.0387 \times 100/1 = 3.87\%$). It would be the recommendation of the author in this situation not to proceed with biopsy but to arrange for review with a repeat PSA in 6 months if the previous profile of the PSA over time is not known.

PSA velocity

The change in the PSA over time offers another approach to enhancing PSA performance as the PSA is likely to rise at a greater rate in the presence of prostate cancer than in those without. If at the time of referral to a specialist the PSA history is known it is helpful to include this in the referral letter. The concept of PSA velocity (PSAV) was first proposed in the early 1990s and it was concluded that a PSA velocity of 0.75 ng/ml/year or greater was predictive of prostate cancer and substantiated the association between advancing cancer and a rising PSA.

From a population-based database of PSA results in men with a PSA < 10 between 1994 and 2003, PSAV had additional value over one PSA value in identifying men with prostate cancer. Many men with prostate cancer might have a 'normal' (< 0.75 ng/ml/year) PSAV. As with total PSA level, there was no PSAV threshold that could reliably predict prostate cancer, but rather a continuum of risk of cancer associated with PSAV level.

Men whose PSA level increases by > 2 ng/ml during the year before the diagnosis of prostate cancer appear to have a relatively high risk of death from prostate cancer (17% at 10 years) despite undergoing radical prostatectomy, compared with those with a rise of < 2 ng/ml (< 5%).

PSA isoforms

Another potential refinement of the PSA utilises the fact that a greater propor- tion of the PSA appears to be in the bound state in patients with prostate cancer. As described earlier part of the circulating PSA is in an inactive unbound form and in benign enlargement a larger proportion of the PSA will be in the unbound form. Therefore, if a 'raised' PSA results from benign enlargement a larger proportion will be in the unbound or free from with a more favourable ratio of the free:total PSA – approximately 20–35% depending on the assay. With a free:total ratio > 25% the risk of prostate cancer is about 10%, but with a free:total ratio of 10% or less this risk rises to 60%.

It is also possible to selectively measure the bound or 'complexed' PSA (cPSA). Although useful, at present these measurements have not replaced total PSA as the first-line test and are only used in secondary care when there is uncertainty about the need for prostate biopsy.

PSA and the management of prostate cancer

Although it is in the controversial areas of diagnosis and screening that PSA has its greatest impact in primary care, PSA has revolutionised the manage- ment of this disease once diagnosed. Serum PSA levels reflect the disease volume and stage, and PSA increases with disease progression falling after successful treatment for prostate cancer.

Staging

It is uncommon for a man with a PSA of < 10 ng/ml to have metastatic prostate cancer and, conversely prostate cancer is usually metastatic if the PSA level is > 100 ng/ml. There is, however, significant overlap in PSA levels between the pathological stages. Investigators have demonstrated significant upstaging following prostatectomy in men with suspected organ confined (T1 or T2) dis- ease, in those with a PSA > 10 ng/ml. If combined with additional parameters, such as degree of abnormality on DRE and the grade of the tumour it can pre-dict pathological stage with a greater degree of accuracy. PSA measurements clearly have a role in identifying patients that require staging with a bone scan. In the absence of bony symptoms a bone scan will rarely demonstrate metas-tases if the PSA is < 20 ng/ml (about 5% of bone scans show metastases in this case).

PSA and progression in active surveillance patients

When expectant management is selected (low-risk disease usually) PSA together with DRE are the principal methods of assessing disease progression. It is usual in the initial stages to monitor the PSA at 3–4 monthly intervals. If the PSA rise is such that the doubling time (PSADT) is < 3 years then it is more likely that the disease is aggressive and given that extended sextant pros-tate biopsies can miss areas of high grade disease it is now recommended that biopsies be repeated after 12–18 months for patients on active surveillance.

PSA following treatment

The PSA test is extraordinarily sensitive at monitoring the response to treat-ment, particularly after radical prostatectomy. The PSA should fall to an undetectable level within six weeks after complete removal of the gland in the absence of residual disease. Most men destined to suffer recurrence do so within two years, and this is important with regard to how long patients should be followed in secondary care. If there are no associated sexual or urinary problems that require specialist management then referral back to primary care would seem reasonable. After radical prostatectomy a PSA > 0.2 ng/ml can be associated with residual or recurrent disease, but this can also be due to small amounts of residual tissue being left behind at the time of surgery (usually at the urethral margin or bladder neck). A rising trend, however, may indicate recurrent disease. A PSA doubling time (PSADT) after radical prostatectomy of less than 9–12 months is correlated with a high risk of metastatic disease. Here PSA is one of the factors used to determine whether a patient should be offered potentially curative second line therapy or hormonal manipulation for palliation.

After external beam radiotherapy, the PSA will decrease after a mean inter-val of one to two years to a value less than 1 ng/ml (the 'nadir' – this is predic-tive of recurrence-free survival). Biochemical recurrence after radiotherapy is defined by an increase of PSA by 2 ng/ml or more above the PSA nadir according to the 2006 Radiation Therapy Oncology Group-American Society for Therapeutic Radiology and Oncology (RTOG-ASTRO) Phoenix Consensus definition, whether or not it is associated with hormonal therapy (medical or surgical castration). Given that hormonal therapy is routinely continued for 2–3 years following radiotherapy the PSA value is also manipulated by endocrine pathways as well as the radiotherapy.

Following the delivery of high-dose radiation to the prostate using permanent I(125) implants inserted under anaesthetic, a benign phenomenon described as PSA bounce can occur; this is defined as a rise of 0.2 ng/ml above an initial PSA nadir with subsequent decline to or below that nadir without treatment.

PSA and hormonal manipulation

After hormonal manipulation, the PSA nadir is correlated with recurrence-free survival. The PSA falls in 80–90% of men started on hormonal treatment and stays low for a mean of 24 to 36 months. A rise in PSA following this corresponds to hormone-independent prostate cancer. The time to hormone independence and the time to reach the nadir have prognostic value for survival.

With improvements in imaging and technology it is likely that in the future that therapy will be directed at focally destroying areas of cancer within the prostate rather than removing or irradiating the whole gland. This has its potential advantages, but will limit the value of PSA because of the PSA produced by residual tissue left untreated.

Key points

- Urinary tract infection, urethral instrumentation, benign prostatic hyperplasia and ejaculation may increase PSA levels, but DRE does not increase the PSA.
- PSA should not be measured without the patient's knowledge and the asymptomatic patient must be fully counselled prior to being offered a PSA test.
- PSA testing is reasonable in men with LUTS but they should be offered an 'opt out' if they so wish.
- The specificity of PSA is increased by considering the age-related ranges and PSA free:total ratios and complexed PSA levels – the latter two tests are usually offered mainly in secondary care.
- PSA is a reliable guide to the stage of disease and response to treatment.

Further reading and bibliography

D'Amico, A. V., Chen, M. H., Roehl, K. A. and Catalona, W. J. (2004) Preoperative PSA velocity and the risk of death from prostate cancer after radical prostatectomy. *N. Engl. J. Med.*, **351**, 125–35.

Parkinson, M. C., Bott, S. R. J., Montironi, R. and Melia, J. (2002) Screening for prostate cancer and its evolution within Britain. *J. Pathol.*, **197**, 139–42.

CHAPTER 14

Prostate cancer – localised disease

Simon Bott, Nitika Silhi and Alison Birtle

Case history

A 52-year-old man comes to see his GP as his brother (58 years of age) has recently been diagnosed with metastatic prostate cancer and has been started on an LHRH (luteinising hormone releasing hormone) analogue. He requests a PSA as he is concerned he may have prostate cancer, which comes back at 9.4 ng/ml. He wishes to know what this means, what will happen next and, if he has cancer, what are his treatment options. His GP discusses the issues with him and then refers him up to his local hospital under their 'two week rule', suggesting that he may well need prostatic biopsies.

History

In the consultation the PSA history should be examined, as previous readings may indicate the speed of rise (PSA velocity) or fluctuations in his PSA reading. A PSA of 9.4 ng/ml gives him a 40% risk of having prostate cancer (at a PSA <4 ng/ml 25% will have prostate cancer; at 4–10 ng/ml 40% have prostate cancer; at > 10 ng/ml 70% have prostate cancer). Symptoms relating to the lower urinary tract should be assessed as advice and treatment may be provided and severe urinary symptoms preclude some oncology treatment such as brachytherapy. Erectile function must be recorded, as this may also impact upon patient preferences for treatment. His past medical history and drug history are relevant; severe co-morbidity may mean that radical therapy for prostate cancer is not warranted, as patients need a life expectancy exceeding 10 years to benefit. A history of inflammatory bowel disease or previous pelvic radiotherapy will exclude external beam radiotherapy. Patients on warfarin need to stop their medication at least five days prior to prostate biopsy and may need to be anticoagulated with heparin, depending on the indication. Aspirin may be safely continued, but clopidogrel is stopped 5–10 days prior to biopsy.

The family history is relevant, as having a single first degree relative with prostate cancer doubles the risk of having prostate cancer, and more than one first degree relative increases the risk by 5–11×.

Examination

Abdominal examination should be performed, particularly to exclude a palpable bladder. A digital rectal examination (DRE) is necessary to assess the size of the prostate and the clinical stage (Table 14.1).

Table 14.1 TNM classification of prostate cancer.

T1	*Impalpable and not visible on imaging*
T1a	Tumour incidental finding in ≤ 5% tissue resected at TURP
T1b	Tumour incidental finding in > 5% tissue resected at TURP
T1c	Tumour identified by needle biopsy
T2	*Tumour confined within the prostate*
T2a	Tumour involves one half of one lobe, or less
T2b	Tumour involves more than one half of one lobe, but not both lobes
T2c	Tumour involves both lobes
T3	*Tumour extends through the prostatic capsule*
T3a	Unilateral or bilateral extracapsular extension
T3b	Tumour invades seminal vesicle(s)
T4	*Tumour is fixed or invades adjacent structures other than the seminal vesicles*: bladder neck, external sphincter, rectum, levator muscles or pelvic wall
N – X, 0, 1	*Lymph nodes* – Not assessed, no regional metastases, regional node metastases
M1 – a, b, c	*Distant metastases* – non-regional lymph node metastases, bone metastases, other site

Investigations (initial)

The GP should perform a dipstick examination of a midstream urine specimen to exclude infection (urinary infection can significantly increase the PSA). If the dipstick is clear the patient will need to be counselled towards having a prostate biopsy. This discussion and the prostatic biopsies themselves are usually performed in secondary care, although the GP should have some knowledge of the benefits and risks of this procedure. The clinician outlines the benefits in terms of making the diagnosis and detecting early prostate cancer when it is still curable, whilst discussing that some prostate cancers do not require treatment. Risks of biopsy are also discussed, including bleeding per urethra and/or per rectum seen in 60–80%, although this is rarely significant (1%) and usually settles in 3–5 days. Haemospermia may also occur and lasts a few weeks – it is of no significance. There is a 1–2% risk of the patient going into urinary retention and a similar number develop severe sepsis following prostate biopsies. We give our patients three doses of Ciprofloxacin to start two hours before their biopsy. A metronidazole suppository is given at the time of biopsy to limit the small risk of an anaerobic infection. Before undergoing prostate biopsy patients are warned of the 10–20% risk of a false negative biopsy and the uncertainties regarding the optimal treatment should prostate cancer be found.

Management and discussion

Prostate cancer is an enigma, being for some one of the most indolent cancers and for others the second biggest male cancer killer in the UK. A male born in the Western world has a 50% lifetime risk of developing prostate cancer (autopsy studies), yet only a 14% risk of being diagnosed, a 6% risk of developing symptoms and a 3% risk of dying from this disease. Incidental tumours are common in post mortem examinations of other solid organs e.g. breast and kidney; however, the high incidence as well as the lack of specificity of the PSA test results in more men being diagnosed with incidental prostate cancer.

Tom Stamey published his seminal work on the potential use of PSA in the diagnosis and management of prostate cancer in 1987. As a result PSA testing became widespread in the UK in the early 1990s. Since then the incidence of prostate cancer has tripled; over 31,000 new cases of prostate cancer are diagnosed in the UK per annum. The increase has largely been due to a greater number of men being diagnosed with low-risk and potentially insignificant tumours. Despite this, prostate cancer is the second leading cause of male cancer death with 10,000 deaths in England and Wales per annum. To put prostate cancer in context, the average five-year survival is 75%; this compares with 81% for breast, 80% for melanoma and 50% for colorectal cancers.

Grading prostate cancer

Prostate cancer is a multifocal disease. A prostate which contains cancer has on average 2–3 separate foci and 7–8 genetically distinct tumours within these foci. Each tumour has its own distinct histopathological appearance and malignant potential. Donald Gleason, in 1966, first described these differing patterns of prostate cancer and in a later study compared these patterns with the outcome of patients in a five-year study of stilboestrol and/or orchidectomy versus placebo. From this work he proposed a grading system whereby the two largest foci of cancer are assigned a grading score from 1–5, and the two scores are added to give a Gleason sum score (e.g. Gleason 3 + 4 = 7). The increase in score indicates a more aggressive high-risk cancer pathologically. Over time modifications have been made; some of the grade 1 and 2 Gleason patterns have been shown to be benign variants and are no longer included. Small volumes of cancer sampled at prostate biopsy under-represent the grade of the whole tumour; consequently nowadays low grade tumours found in prostate biopsies are all grouped as Gleason sum score 6. There is a tendency for low grade tumours found in prostate biopsies to be up-graded when the whole tumour is examined after radical prostatectomy, in 40–50% of cases. Likewise, a third of high grade tumours in biopsies will be downgraded if the whole tumour is examined. This arises as processing of the biopsy tissue may compress the prostate glands, giving them the appearance of sheets of cancer cells, a characteristic of high grade disease, rather than the genuine glandular structure seen in lower grade disease. Despite its limitations the Gleason grading system remains the most useful prognostic marker in prostate cancer management.

Localised prostate cancer

Localised prostate cancer is cancer that is confined to the prostate, or T2 or less (TNM classification, Table 14.1) and 58% of men diagnosed with prostate cancer in the UK present with this potentially curable localised disease.

The position of the prostate within the pelvis and its close relationship with important adjacent structures complicates curative treatment. From a surgical perspective there is little surrounding fascia to take with the specimen to enhance the chance of resection margins clear of tumour. Furthermore, vital structures are in close proximity; the external urethral sphincter (integral to urinary continence) lies just distal to the prostatic apex, the thin Denonvillier's fascia posteriorly separates the prostate and the rectum, and the trigone of the bladder abuts the prostatic base. The close proximity of these structures not only restricts cancer clearance surgically, but also gives rise to the side effects experienced by some men after all radical treatments.

To compound matters there is no preoperative examination or test that accurately predicts whether clinically localised prostate cancer is confined to the prostate pathologically. The three best investigations, namely the preoperative PSA, the Gleason grade of cancer at biopsy and the proportion of prostatic biopsy cores invaded with cancer are often combined and fed into predictive tables: for example the PCUK tables (http://www.baus.org.uk/). These give an individual the likelihood that his cancer is organ confined, extraprostatic or metastatic based on a large series of UK men. Improvements are being made in imaging technologies, including PET/CT and MRI; currently accuracy rates in excess of 80% are reported with these techniques, but their widespread use is currently not advocated for the majority of patients.

Men diagnosed with clinically localised prostate cancer have three main options: radical surgery (open, laparoscopic or robotic prostatectomy), radical radiotherapy (external beam or brachytherapy) and active surveillance. In some areas in the UK, as part of a clinical trial high-energy focused ultrasound (HIFU) may also be offered.

A landmark Scandinavian study randomised nearly 700 men to radical prostatectomy versus a watch and wait policy (refer to the paper by Bill-Axelson *et al.* in Further reading). At ten years there was a significant difference in disease-free survival (DFS) of 44% and an overall survival (OS) of 26% in favour of radical prostatectomy. The absolute risk reductions however were modest (5% DFS, 5% OS). This translates to needing to treat 20 men with radical prostatectomy for 1 man to benefit by 10 years.

Unfortunately, this study raised as many questions as it answered and highlights some of the issues in prostate cancer trials. On the one hand, benefit in terms of disease free and overall survival was seen in a small number of men undergoing radical prostatectomy compared with watch and wait. Furthermore, improvements in the prevention of local progression and development of metastatic disease were even greater in the surgical arm. Radical prostatectomy is undertaken in men with a life expectancy exceeding 10 years, as the benefits of surgery are greatest beyond this period. The longer-term results are likely to show an increase in benefit from surgery as the greater number of men in the watch and wait arm who have developed local and metastatic progression succumb to their advancing disease. On the other hand, as this study recruited from 1989, the patient mix contained men who were older than most current series (64.7 years compared with 58 years in recent series), and their patients had higher PSA levels and higher clinical stage disease than contemporary series. What is more, nearly 10% of patients randomised actually opted for the opposite treatment.

This study emphasises the problems of performing adequate trials comparing the various treatment options in localised prostate cancer. As the disease has a protracted course, by the time valid data have been accrued the population investigated is no longer representative of current practice. Furthermore, as a large amount of un-randomised data has been available on the outcomes of treatment for a number of years, randomly allocating patients a treatment against the background of this information is problematic.

Further study results, including the UK ProtecT study in which men with PSA screen detected tumours are randomised to receive surgery, external beam radiotherapy or active surveillance, are awaited. In the meantime the decision is based on the nature of the cancer at biopsy – Gleason grade, number and site of cores involved, the PSA, the patient's co-morbid status and careful discussion between healthcare professionals as well as with the individual and his family.

Treatment options for localised disease

Radical prostatectomy

Radical prostatectomy involves the removal of the entire prostate, seminal vesicles and frequently the obturator lymph nodes, the latter for staging purposes. It may be performed via the retropubic approach, either through a small (6–10 cm) incision, or increasingly using a laparoscopic or robotic technique. Alternatively, and less commonly, the perineal approach may be employed. The incidence of tumour at the resection limit (a positive surgical margin) is similar for each technique, but the location of the limits is dependent upon the approach, and nowadays should be 10–20%, depending on patient selection.

Laparoscopic prostatectomy is a technically demanding procedure and there is a significant learning curve. Nevertheless, this technique, sometimes aided by a robot, is becoming increasingly popular as the postoperative hospital stay is 2–4 days compared with 4–6 days after the conventional approach. Furthermore, as the anastomosis between the bladder and urethral stump is performed under magnification, urinary continence may resume earlier. The robot is reported to reduce the learning curve whilst maintaining the benefits of a shorter recovery time seen with the laparoscopic approach. Clearly cost and availability currently restrict robotic radical prostatectomy to a few centres in the UK, though these are increasing year on year.

Whichever route is taken the disease-specific outcomes are similar. Cancer cure rates at 10 years after radical surgery are in excess of 80% of men in the American series. Most men in North America are diagnosed by PSA screening and probably present earlier in the disease course. In the UK, two studies have reported outcomes similar to this, albeit with short follow-up (2–3 years).

One of the advantages of excising the prostate is that the serum PSA should fall to an undetectable level within a month of surgery. Regular follow-up, including PSA checks, can detect recurrent disease eight years before metastases develop, and if metastases develop, a further five years before death from prostate cancer. In the event of a PSA rise further treatments can be offered with potentially curative intent. This includes external beam radiotherapy to the prostate bed if local recurrence is suspected or palliative treatment with hormonal manipulation if systemic disease is diagnosed.

Side effects of radical prostatectomy

In 1982 Walsh and Donker published their seminal work on the anatomy of the dorsal venous complex and the cavernosal nerves (the latter promote erection). An understanding of the site of the blood vessels enables better intraoperative bleeding control; this improves vision and allows more accurate dissection around the urethral sphincter, which is essential for urinary continence. Continence rates, defined as 'pad free', are as high as 95% in most large centres now, although a proportion of men may suffer stress incontinence for a few weeks after surgery.

Walsh and Donker's observation that the cavernosal (erectile) nerves run alongside the prostate, rather than within the capsule, means that in many men the nerves can safely be left intact improving the chance of post-operative potency. The decision on whether to preserve one or both erectile nerve bundles depends on the site and extent of disease at biopsy, as well as preoperative erectile function. Prostate cancer has a tendency to invade perineural spaces and the short inferior neurovascular pedicle at the apex renders extraprostatic extension more common at this site. In men with extensive apical cancers (the most common site) or high-grade disease, it may be appropriate to sacrifice one or both erectile nerve bundles, and potentially potency, in order to achieve cancer cure. In the majority of men though, one or both nerve bundles can be left intact without jeopardising the important goal of total cancer clearance. In the best hands, potency can be preserved in up to 80% of men, though this will depend on the age of the patient, the stage of disease and the number of nerve bundles left intact at the end of the operation. Men troubled by erectile dysfunction after surgery usually benefit from oral therapies, such as tadalafil, sildenafil or vardenafil; alternatively intraurethral or intracavernosal alprostadil may be used.

External beam radiotherapy (EBRT)

Standard external beam radiotherapy offers men with clinically localised disease an alternative to surgery, with similar efficacy but with differing complications. Megavoltage radiotherapy has been available for over 40 years, but new techniques are developing rapidly. CT planning allows a clearer assessment of the prostate and surrounding normal tissues. In general, one outpatient planning session is required prior to starting treatment, which is performed daily on weekdays, over a 4–7½ week period. The radiation dose is limited by the tolerance of normal tissue in the irradiated area and UK doses should be at least 74 Gray or its biologically equivalent dose. Radiation fractionation trials such as ChHIP assessing improved cancer control and improved side effects are ongoing.

Cancer control rates as defined as a PSA of < 2 ng/ml at two years after treatment are between 35% and 80% with standard external beam radiotherapy. These rates can be improved by increasing the dose of radiotherapy – dose escalation – such that a 10% increase in dose may improve local control by up to 20%. Conformal radiotherapy, provides both dose escalation and better tumour control. This technique allows the irradiated volume to be shaped to match the irregular prostate volume/outline, reducing the normal tissue treated and thereby the dose-limiting side effects from 15% to 5%. Dose escalation appears to benefit particularly men with higher-grade disease (Gleason grade 8–10).

A further modification of radiotherapy is intensity-modulated radiotherapy (IMRT), where differing doses of radiation are given across the irradiated volume, sparing normal structures and delivering higher doses to the tumour. Cancer control using IMRT is expected to be superior to conventional radiotherapy; however, data on cancer outcomes is not yet mature.

Standard radiotherapy treatment now includes a period of three months of luteinising hormone releasing hormone (LHRH) agonist prior to radiotherapy. This allows for the tumour to shrink (cytoreduction), enabling smaller volumes to be treated and so reducing the amount of normal tissue that is irradiated. In addition, a significant difference in local failure rates (32% vs. 43% at eight years in the treated and untreated, respectively) and the progression-free survival has been demonstrated in poor prognosis patients receiving radiotherapy.

Several large studies have confirmed the benefit of at least two years of adjuvant LHRH agonist therapy subsequent to radical radiotherapy for patients with high grade (Gleason score 8–10) tumours. Significant advantages in disease-specific survival and overall survival were seen with a median follow-up of over five years.

Acute side effects as a result of 'normal tissue' exposure usually start towards the end of the fourth week of treatment and peak 10 days after completing radiotherapy. These include diarrhoea, managed with a low fibre diet and loperamide, tenesmus and proctitis. Proctosedyl suppositories may be of benefit for the latter symptom. A high fluid intake is recommended to reduce urinary side effects, namely dysuria and frequency. Lethargy is also experienced, especially towards the end of treatment, though this and the other acute side effects usually settle within six weeks of completing radiotherapy.

Side effects occurring more than three months after the end of radiotherapy are termed 'late side effects' and may include impotence in 10–30% of men. This may be confounded by the use of adjuvant hormonal therapy, albeit usually temporarily. Incontinence is very unusual and disturbance in stool frequency and consistency occurs in less than 20% of men. A small minority of men develop chronic proctitis, giving rise to bleeding and fibrosis, with a 1–2% risk of surgical intervention. Bowel complications persisting for more than six months require further investigation to exclude an underlying bowel neoplasm. Following prostate radiotherapy there is a 1.5–2 times increased risk of secondary tumours in the large bowel and bladder. Recent guidance suggests that men should be offered sigmoidoscopy every five years after prostate radiotherapy to detect these tumours.

Many patients will also be receiving an LHRH agonist, and these are associated with side effects. These include hot flushes, loss of libido and erectile dysfunction, breast enlargement and pain, cognitive impairment and (if prolonged) a decrease in bone mineral density. Hot flushes may be treated with cyproterone acetate 50 mg od; the other side effects may improve on cessation of hormonal therapy, although this can take up to 12 months.

Brachytherapy

This involves the insertion of a radioactive source directly into the prostate, allowing a high dose of radiation to be delivered over short distance around the source, sparing normal tissue. Two types are used in the treatment of localised prostate cancer: iodine 125 seeds as a permanent low-dose implant, and iridium 192 as a temporary high-dose implant, used in conjunction with external beam radiotherapy. The selection criteria are different for both types of treatment and brachytherapy is only available in a few specialist centres.

Iodine 125 seeds

To be considered for seed brachytherapy patients must have a life expectancy exceeding 10 years, clinically localised cancer of Gleason grade 7 or less, a low prostate volume (< 50 ml) and no previous prostate surgery. A transrectal ultrasound is performed to assess prostate volume and to plan treatment. Subsequently 20–30 needles are implanted via the perineum using ultrasound guidance. The needles contain up to 120 seeds in total, depending on prostate size and seed activity. The patient receives a spinal or general anaesthetic and is usually in hospital overnight. The largest study with 12-year data showed that 87% of these 'good prognosis' men were PSA free at 10 years.

Complications occur as a result of radiation damage to the urethra and include both storage and voiding urinary symptoms, which may last for a few months but return to baseline by nine months after seed implantation. Incontinence rates are reported as < 1%, rising to 50% in men who have had a transurethral resection of the prostate for benign hyperplasia; hence these patients are now excluded from brachytherapy. Erectile dysfunction rates are similar to radical prostatectomy, although they take up to five years to develop after prostate brachytherapy.

High-dose iridium 192 rods

These are used in men with more unfavourable disease: PSA > 10 ng/ml or Gleason score 8–10. They provide a radiation boost and are used in conjunction with a 4½-week course of external beam radiotherapy. Hollow rods are positioned in the prostate using ultrasound guidance with the patient under spinal or general anaesthesia. The patient receives three separate doses with a minimum of six hours between each dose. The rods remain *in situ* throughout the treatment, so the patient is kept in the lithotomy position for at least 18 hours. Unsurprisingly, backache is a common complaint with this treatment.

The side effects, including incontinence and erectile dysfunction, are similar to EBRT, with the added complication associated with the anaesthetic. There is also a risk of urethral stricture in 6% of men. Despite this, excellent PSA free rates of 79–89% at five years have been reported in these men with less favourable disease.

Active surveillance

Active surveillance involves observing a patient's prostate cancer with regular PSA measurements and repeated prostate biopsies and initiating radical treatment should progression occur. One schedule for active surveillance includes men with Gleason < 3 + 4, and less than 50% biopsy cores involved, organ-confined disease and total PSA < 15 ng/ml. Patients are followed with three-monthly PSA checks during the first year and re-biopsy of the prostate at 12–24 months, with indications for radical treatment being upgraded pathology on re-biopsy, change in PSA by > 1 ng/ml/year, change in clinical stage or patient preference. Clearly this approach is fundamentally different from the traditional approach of infrequent PSA monitoring and no further biopsies in the patient managed by watchful waiting. In addition, as for all radical treatment options for localised prostate cancer, the patient requires a predicted ten-year life expectancy. Active surveillance has been recently recommended as the favoured treatment option for men with low and intermediate risk prostate cancer by NICE. However, these guidelines have been criticised for drawing definitive conclusions where evidence is lacking. Indeed, the optimal protocol for the frequency of PSA testing and repeat biopsy is not known. Furthermore the rate of rise in an individual's PSA is an unreliable predictor of disease progression. Reported studies use differing criteria for disease progression including rate of PSA rise, Gleason up-grading or number and volume of biopsy cores invaded by tumour. The studies are too small and have too short follow-up for a sufficient number of events to have occurred. Therefore meaningful conclusions in terms of which factors best predict oncological outcome are not established.

This said, clearly a large number of men do not need active treatment of their prostate cancer. Active surveillance series report a prostate cancer mortality rate of 1–2% with eight-year follow-up, and 20–30% of men receive radical treatment, either because of disease progression or because patients change their minds. Concerns about patient anxiety each time they have a PSA test as part of the surveillance process seem unfounded, at least in men who chose this 'treatment' plan. Active surveillance remains a treatment option for patients with low risk and (in some series) intermediate risk groups, as shown in Table 14.2. In addition, potential new markers and chemoprevention agents can be studied in this group of patients who are undergoing planned repeat biopsies. Nevertheless, it remains only one of a number of choices for patients with organ-confined disease and a full discussion of all treatment options is mandatory.

Traditional watchful waiting is considered in men with low grade low volume prostate cancer whose age or co-morbidities mean that they are more likely to die of causes other than their organ-confined prostate cancer. For these patients, a three- to six-monthly follow-up schedule with treatment implemented when symptoms intervene is recommended, and many patients can safely be managed in the primary care setting.

Table 14.2 Complication rates after curative treatment for localised prostate cancer.

Complication	Radical prostatectomy	External beam radiotherapy	Brachytherapy
Death	0–2%	NA	NA
Incontinence	0–15%	5%	0–19%
Erectile dysfunction	20–100%	10–30%	14–38%
Rectal injury/ bleeding	< 1%	20%	1–21%
Urinary retention	NA	< 1%	1–10%

High-intensity focused ultrasound (HIFU)

High-intensity focused ultrasound is a technique which has been employed in prostate cancer and benign prostatic hyperplasia for over a decade. Despite this, long-term outcome data are not currently available. For this reason HIFU is considered an experimental procedure and patients undergoing HIFU should all be enlisted on a national database so that results are available for medical and wider public scrutiny.

HIFU is considered less invasive, with a lower incidence of side effects compared with traditional radical treatments. It may therefore be more appropriate for older men (> 72 years) or men with lower risk disease who want treatment but not the side effects of radical treatments. HIFU may also be offered to men in whom prostate radiotherapy is contraindicated, including inflammatory bowel disease or previous pelvic radiation.

HIFU involves a single procedure, under general anaesthetic. An ultrasound probe is inserted into the rectum; this generates real-time images of the prostate, as well as generating a treatment ultrasound wave. The imaging is used to plan the treatment and continually assess the prostate during the treatment. The focused ultrasound heats a volume of prostate the size of a rice grain sequentially. Cell death occurs above 60 °C; HIFU heats the prostate to 70–90 °C in 3 seconds, resulting in coagulative necrosis. Patients are usually discharged on the day of treatment with a urethral or suprapubic catheter. In patients without a satisfactory PSA response or a rising PSA after treatment, HIFU can be repeated, without any significant worsening of side effects.

Similar to other non-invasive treatments of the prostate the definition of disease relapse is problematic. The PSA does not fall to undetectable levels, so a PSA nadir of < 0.1 up to < 1.0 ng/ml has been used. At three years follow-up

60–80% achieve a PSA below a nadir. In some reported series prostate biopsies are performed several months following treatment; between 80% and 95% of these biopsies show no viable tumour. The equipment is being updated all the time, so these results are likely to improve. In the meantime, prostate HIFU remains an experimental treatment and patients should be made aware of this before undergoing treatment.

Conclusions

The ageing population and the increasing awareness of PSA and prostate cancer mean that the number of men requiring treatment for prostate cancer will continue to rise. Patients with localised disease now have a choice of treatments ranging from active surveillance in low-risk disease to radical surgery or combined EBRT and adjuvant hormonal therapy in more high-risk disease. There is a pressing need for more sensitive markers of prostate cancer progression. This will better enable men with potentially life-threatening disease to undergo the best cancer curing procedure whilst safely deferring treatment in those with less aggressive prostate cancer.

Key points

- Patients who have a raised PSA, in the absence of urinary infection, should be counselled to have prostate biopsies.
- A male born in the Western world has a 50% lifetime risk of developing prostate cancer (autopsy studies), yet only a 14% risk of being diagnosed, a 6% risk of developing symptoms and a 3% risk of dying from this disease.
- Localised prostate cancer is cancer that is confined to the prostate, or T2 or less (TNM classification) and 58% of men diagnosed with prostate cancer in the UK present with this potentially curable localised disease.
- The options for localised prostate disease include active surveillance, radical prostatectomy (open, laparoscopic, robotic), radical external beam conformal radiotherapy and brachytherapy, and (in a trial setting) high-intensity focused ultrasound is being increasingly used.
- The appropriate management option in localised disease is decided by the pathology of the disease and after careful discussion between health professionals and the patient.

Further reading and biliography

Stamey, T. A., Yang, N., Hay, A. R., McNeal, J. E., Freiha, F. S. and Redwine, E. (1987) Prostate-specific antigen as a serum marker for adenocarcinoma of the prostate. *N. Engl. J. Med.*, **317**, 909–16.

Bill-Axelson, A., Holmberg, L., Ruutu, M., Haggman, M., Andersson, S. O., Bratell, S. *et al.* (2005) Radical prostatectomy versus watchful waiting in early prostate cancer. *N. Engl. J. Med.*, **352**, 1977–84.

Pound, C. R., Partin, A. W., Eisenberger, M. A., Chan, D. W., Pearson, J. D. and Walsh, P. C. (1999) Natural history of progression after PSA elevation following radical prostatectomy. *JAMA*, **281**, 1591–7.

Horwich, A., Wynne, C., Nahum, A., Swindell, W. and Dearnaley, D. P. (1994) Conformal radiotherapy at the Royal Marsden Hospital (UK). *Int. J. Radiat. Biol.*, **65**, 117–22.

Martinez, A. A., Gustafson, G., Gonzalez, J., Armour, E., Mitchell, C., Edmundson, G. *et al.* (2002) Dose escalation using conformal high-dose-rate brachytherapy improves outcome in unfavorable prostate cancer. *Int. J. Radiat. Oncol. Biol. Phys.*, **53**, 316–27.

Nobes, J. P., Wells, I. G., Khaksar, S. J., Money-Kyrle, J. F., Laing, R. W. and Langley, S. E. (2008) Biochemical relapse-free survival in 400 patients treated with I-125 prostate brachytherapy: the Guildford experience. *Prostate Cancer Prostatic Dis Advance* online publication Apr 22 2008; doi; 10.1038/pcan.2008.17.

CHAPTER 15

Prostate cancer – locally advanced and metastatic disease

Simon Bott, Nitika Silhi and Alison Birtle

Case history

A 78-year-old man presents to his GP with a three-month history of worsening lumbar back pain. He has lost a stone in weight and is having increasing difficulty passing urine. His GP performs a digital rectal examination which reveals a hard nodular prostate, requests a number of blood tests (including a PSA), gives him some oral analgesia and asks him to return to the practice in three days for the results. On his return the patient complains that over the last 24 hours he has had increasing difficulty walking as his right leg gives way. The PSA has come back at 854 ng/ml. The GP is concerned that the patient has metastatic prostate cancer to the vertebral column, resulting in spinal cord compression and refers him directly to the on-call urology service.

History

In this situation a history of worsening lower urinary tract symptoms indicates either locally advanced disease encroaching/obstructing the urethra or, more worryingly, compression of the spinal cord at the S2, 3, 4 level by metastatic disease affecting the efferent nerve supply to the bladder (and thus the bladder not emptying). A history of leg weakness, loss of sensation or constipation helps confirm cord compression.

Examination

Abdominal examination should be performed to exclude a palpable bladder. A rectal examination will confirm prostate malignancy, and also abnormalities in the anal tone and ano-cutaneous reflex would point to spinal cord compression at S2–S4 level (by metastatic deposits in vertebrae). Lower limb neurological examination is essential in this case.

Investigations

A PSA level and an urgent MRI of the spine, to confirm the diagnosis and identify the level of cord compression, are mandatory. Isotope bone scan will also show metastatic deposits in other regions.

Management and discussion

Cord compression occurs in up to 10% of men with metastatic prostate cancer. *It requires immediate treatment to prevent the devastating development of paraplegia and loss of urinary and bowel control.*

The initial management includes high-dose intravenous steroids (dexamethasone). The cord compression is usually treated first with either urgent radiotherapy, surgical decompression with laminectomy or combined treatment. It is essential that discussion with an oncologist and/or neurosurgeon occurs at the earliest opportunity, as the most effective recovery is seen when patients are treated within 24 hours of the onset of symptoms. Androgen deprivation therapy is used first line to treat metastatic prostate cancer; but in this case where *rapid* castrate levels are required an orchidectomy (bilateral) was offered.

This gentleman was started on steroids and an MRI confirmed sclerotic bone metastases with cord compression. Radiotherapy was planned for the following day and he was consented for a bilateral subcapsular orchidectomy. In this procedure only the contents of the testis are removed, leaving the tunica albuginea (outer covering of testis). This means the patient still has visible, albeit slightly smaller, testes. Symptomatic improvement was seen after he completed palliative radiotherapy and he was discharged home on a reducing dose of dexamethasone, with planned early urological clinic follow-up.

Advanced prostate cancer

The management of advanced prostatic cancer, like localised disease, depends on tumour characteristics – including the histological Gleason grade, clinical and radiological stage of disease, and the prostate specific antigen (PSA) level. This together with the patient's chronological and biological age and co-morbidities is considered and facilitates a multidisciplinary team approach. Advanced prostate cancer may be divided into locally advanced and metastatic disease.

Locally advanced prostate cancer

In the UK, locally advanced prostate cancers account for 40% of prostate cancers at presentation. These include carcinomas where one or two acini (glands) have penetrated through the prostatic capsule to those bulky tumours invading adjacent structures, such as the bladder trigone, rectum, urethra and the pelvic side wall. Therapeutic options include external beam radiotherapy (EBRT) (with or without neoadjuvant or adjuvant androgen ablation), surgery in selected cases, androgen ablation alone or active monitoring.

External beam radiotherapy (EBRT) and androgen ablation

For patients with minimal co-morbities and locally advanced disease, radical external beam radiotherapy is an option. Three months of neoadjuvant therapy with a luteinising hormone releasing hormone (LHRH) analogue is followed by radical radiotherapy for up to 7.5 weeks. LHRH therapy is continued during and for three years following radiotherapy. This prolonged adjuvant treatment offers a significant improvement in both metastatic and biochemical relapse rates and overall survival when compared to only a short course of androgen ablation (with LHRH agonists) given immediately prior to and during radiotherapy.

Androgen ablation involves chemical castration with LHRH analogues or surgical orchidectomy. However, reduced libido and increased fatigue are often associated with both these treatments. Non-steroidal anti-androgen monotherapy with bicalutamide 150 mg once daily for T3/T4 disease, compared with LHRH agonists has been evaluated. No significant difference has been seen between the two types of drug in terms of overall survival and time to progression, although significant improvements in sexual interest and physical capacity were reported with bicalutamide. Bicalutamide also improves bone mineral density, contrasting with the 3–6.5% loss per annum seen in patients on long-term LHRH analogues, albeit at the expense of increased gynaeco-mastia and breast tenderness.

For selected patients with locally advanced T3 disease, high-dose rate iridium brachytherapy together with a shortened course of pelvic EBRT, as described for poor risk localised prostate cancer, may be considered, to allow dose escalation and improvement of local control rates.

Radical prostatectomy

For younger men with low-volume extraprostatic disease radical prostatec-tomy may be offered. A third of men undergoing surgery are found to have disease confined to the prostate as a result of staging inaccuracies at the time of diagnosis; clearly these men will benefit from surgery. In experienced hands a wider resection margin can be taken to improve the likelihood of total cancer clearance. In the event of poor risk findings at pathological examination of the prostatectomy specimen, adjuvant radiotherapy has been shown to improve the PSA-free survival but not disease-specific survival, and is not used routinely.

For asymptomatic patients over 70 years old with low grade disease, active monitoring may be a favoured option. Although a significant survival advan-tage in those having immediate hormonal therapy (versus delayed hormonal treatment) was initially thought to be best practice, subsequent follow-up of patients has shown much less of a survival difference and thus the potential benefits and side-effects of early androgen deprivation treatment warrant a full discussion with the patient.

Intermittent hormone therapy

Intermittent hormone therapy may used in the treatment of both locally advanced and metastatic disease. It has been known for some time that patients who stop androgen ablative treatments may have a period of time being symptom free from their prostate cancer and side effects of treatment. Furthermore, they usually respond again to first line therapy at the time of relapse, deferring the time to the development of hormone-resistant disease. In locally advanced but asymptomatic recurrent disease, men have a median survival of 7–8 years, and long-term hor-monal therapy may negatively impact on their quality of life. We recommend an initial eight months of treatment with androgen ablation and then a variable period of time off treatment, recommencing when the PSA is greater than 10 ng/ml or 20 ng/ml. This intermittent therapy may well prolong treatment time as well as reduce the incidence of side effects during the off treatment periods. However, results of trials are awaited before intermittent therapy becomes routine.

Metastatic prostate cancer

Androgen ablation

The first line treatment in a man with symptomatic metastatic prostate cancer is androgen ablation by medical (LHRH agonists) or surgical castration (bilateral subcapsular orchidectomy). This has an initial PSA response rate of around 85%, maintained for on average 18–24 months. No difference in efficacy has been seen between orchidectomy and the use of the LHRH agonists, though the incidence of side effects may be lower in the orchidectomy group. Patient choice, age and co-morbidity determine which option is favoured.

The initiation of an LHRH agonist results in a tumour flare – this is inhibited by using a peripheral anti-androgen (bicalutamide, flutamide, cyproterone acetate) for three days prior to and for three weeks following the initiation of an LHRH analogue. The side effects of chemical castration include erectile dysfunction, reduced libido, tiredness, sweating, hot flushes, weight gain, breast changes and anaemia.

Although immediate hormonal therapy has shown only a negligible survival benefit in the asymptomatic patient with metastases, there is certainly evidence of a reduction in important complications, including the incidence of spinal cord compression and ureteric obstruction.

Options when first line treatment with LHRH analogues fails (i.e. cancer becomes hormone refractory)

After initiation of LHRH analogues, prostate cancer can become resistant to this treatment at a mean of about four years. Recurrence after this first line hormonal therapy with an LHRH agonist (indicated by a rising PSA) reflects a poor outlook, with a mean survival of 2–3 years. The development of newer agents, however, means that selected patients can have durable responses to treatment. Choices of therapy include maximum androgen blockade, oral or dermal oestrogens, low-dose steroids (prednisolone, dexamethasone) or chemotherapy.

- **Maximum androgen blockade**: surgical (subcapsular orchidectomy) or medical castration (LHRH analogue) is known to reduce circulating testosterone levels by ~90% (this testosterone is secreted by the testes). The remaining 10% of testosterone is secreted by the adrenals. In an attempt to reduce the action of adrenal testosterone, peripheral antagonists, such as bicalutamide/flutamide/cyproterone acetate (anti-androgens), may be added to an LHRH agonist. The outcome of this combined androgen block-ade (maximum androgen blockade) remains unclear, as there is conflict-ing data, although meta-analyses suggest the benefit to be of the order of 1–2%, predominantly in patients with low metastatic load and good per-formance status.

■ **Oestrogens**: stilboestrol 1 mg is widely used in the UK and has shown effective clinical response rates of around 66% in patients with one previ-ous hormonal manipulation and 13% in those with two or more. However, an increase in thromboembolic and cardiovascular side effects is seen and concurrent low-dose anticoagulation with warfarin or aspirin is in common use. The cardiovascular side effects associated with oestrogen therapy are due to clotting factors generated by the metabolism of oestrogens during their first passage through the liver. An interesting newer method of admin-istering oestrogens is the use of intramuscular polyoestradiol phosphate (PEP) or hormone replacement therapy patches. The first pass effect is avoided, reducing the risk of cardiovascular events. Prophylactic nipple radiation may be given to reduce the incidence of gynaecomastia seen in patients on oestrogens.

■ **Steroids**: prednisolone started after failure of first line hormonal therapy has elicited subjective symptomatic response rates of 56% compared with a 46% response rate to flutamide. There was also a biochemical response rate (lowering of PSA level) of 21% and 23% respectively, but no difference in overall survival between the two groups. Low dose dexamethasone has a response rate of ~50% with median duration of response of seven months.

■ **Chemotherapy for metastatic disease**: the use of chemotherapy in hor-mone refractory metastatic prostate cancer is the subject of many ongoing studies. The license for taxotere for use in hormone refractory prostate cancer in 2004 significantly increased the role of chemotherapy in this patient group. It has been demonstrated that three-weekly taxotere with prednisolones is associated with improved survival outcomes, reduced pain and better quality of life. Taxotere is now standard of care for patients with hormone-resistant prostate cancer of good performance status.

Radiotherapy

Local radiotherapy may be useful for perineal pain, bleeding or bone pain. Any metastasis in a weight-bearing bone requires plain X-ray review to assess the cortical integrity, and orthopaedic assessment if > 50% of the cortex is affected, to determine whether prophylactic stabilisation is required. Local radiation may be offered as an alternative if the patient is unfit for surgical intervention. A single fraction of local radiotherapy is effective for pain relief in symptomatic bony metastases in up to 75% of patients. It may, however, take several weeks before its effect is manifest. Hemibody irradiation is utilised where a large treatment field is required, usually encompassing the pelvis and the upper femurs; however, this frequently results in diarrhoea and nausea.

Strontium 89 as an intravenous injection may be used for pain control in widespread bony metastases. It may be associated with an initial pain flare but approximately 10% of treated patients do experience a complete resolution of pain. However, the presence of any critical metastases potentially able to cause spinal cord compression must be excluded, as strontium may cause oedema at these sites. In addition, the treatment commonly produces prolonged myelosuppression, particularly thrombocytopenia, and in patients with already depleted marrow reserves, due to either disease or treatment, this can be problematic. It may also limit future treatment options, such as chemotherapy, because of its side effects.

Bisphosphonates in metastatic prostate cancer

Bone complications in prostate cancer occur as a result of skeletal metastases, long-term treatment with androgen withdrawal and following radiotherapy. Bisphosphonates, now widely used in breast cancer, have been shown to reduce bone pain in prostatic cancer for 2–3 weeks after a single intravenous infusion in up to 30% of patients, and are in widespread use for symptomatic patients. Bisphophonates act by decreasing the rate of bone turnover, reducing the number of osteoclasts, their recruitment, lifespan and activity The use of prophylactic zoledronic acid (15 minute infusion of every three weeks), the most potent bisphosphonate, has been shown to decrease the total number and the time to the first skeletal event in those patients with metastases. Questions remain about the importance of all the skeletal related events, such as asymptomatic vertebral crush fractures. Bisphosphonates did not have a significant impact on individual events or on patients' overall quality of life. Therefore, their use in men with asymptomatic bone metastases remains to be clearly defined.

Conclusions

Some men with low-volume extraprostatic disease may be cured with either radical surgery or external beam radiotherapy in combination with androgen withdrawal. Men with more extensive locally advanced and metastatic disease can be treated successfully, allowing disease control for a finite period of time before eventual disease relapse. Taxotere-based chemotherapy is standard treatment in appropriately selected patients of good performance status. Zoledronic acid improves symptoms from bone metastases but its use as a disease modifier is controversial. Further developments in our understanding of the genetics of this disease will allow the identification of new molecular markers and novel therapeutic targets.

Key points

- In locally advanced (not metastatic) prostate cancer therapeutic options include external beam radiotherapy (with or without neo-adjuvant or adjuvant androgen ablation), surgery in selected cases, androgen ablation alone (either LHRH agonist or monotherapy with bicalutamide) or active monitoring.
- The first line treatment in a man with symptomatic metastatic prostate cancer is androgen ablation by medical (LHRH agonists) or surgical castration (bilateral subcapsular orchidectomy).
- The initiation of an LHRH agonist results in a tumour flare – this is inhibited by using a peripheral anti-androgen (bicalutamide, flutamide, cyproterone acetate) for three days prior to and for three weeks following the initiation of an LHRH analogue.
- After initiation of LHRH analogues, prostate cancer can become resistant to this treatment (hormone-resistant prostate cancer) at a mean of about four years. Choices of therapy in this situation include maximum androgen blockade (LHRH analogue plus anti-androgen such as bicalutamide/flutamide/cyproterone acetate), oral or dermal oestrogens, low dose steroids (prednisolone, dexamethasone) or chemotherapy.
- Spinal cord compression occurs in up to 10% of men with metastatic prostate cancer. It requires immediate treatment to prevent the devastating development of paraplegia and loss of urinary and bowel control.

Further reading and bibliography

Berthold, D. R., Pond, G. R., Soban, F., de Wit, R., Eisenberger, M. and Tannock, I. F. (2008) Docetaxel plus prednisone or mitoxantrone plus prednisone for advanced prostate cancer: updated survival in the TAX 327 study. *J. Clin. Oncol.*, **26**, 242–5.

Bolla, M., Gonzalez, D., Warde, P., Dubois, J. B., Mirimanoff, R. O., Storme, G. *et al.* (1997) Improved survival in patients with locally advanced prostate cancer treated with radiotherapy and goserelin. *N. Engl. J. Med.*, **337**, 295–300.

Medical Research Council Prostate Cancer Working Party Investigators Group. Immediate versus deferred treatment for advanced prostatic cancer: initial results of the Medical Research Council Trial. *Br. J. Urol.*, **79**, 235–46.

Prostate Cancer Trialists' Collaborative Group (1995) Maximum androgen blockade in advanced prostate cancer: an overview of 22 randomised trials with 3283 deaths in 5710 patients. *Lancet*, **346**, 265–9.

Robinson, M. R., Smith, P. H., Richards, B., Newling, D. W., de Pauw, M. and Sylvester, R. (1995) The final analysis of the EORTC Genito-Urinary Tract Cancer Co-Operative Group phase III clinical trial (protocol 30805) comparing orchidectomy, orchidectomy plus cyproterone acetate and low dose stilboestrol in the management of metastatic carcinoma of the prostate. *Eur. Urol.*, **28**, 273–83.

Saad, F., Gleason, D. M., Murray, R., Tchekmedyian, S., Venner, P., Lacombe, L. *et al.* (2002) A randomized, placebo-controlled trial of zoledronic acid in patients with hormone-refractory metastatic prostate carcinoma. *J. Natl. Cancer Inst.*, **94**, 1458–68.

PART II

Paediatric urology

CHAPTER 16

The prepuce: normal development, phimosis and circumcision

Nilay Patel, Vinay Kalsi, Asif Muneer, Nitika Silhi and Imran Mushtaq

Case history

A fit and well 18-month-old boy presents to the surgery with a non-retractile foreskin. His parents have also noticed that the prepuce balloons upon micturition. He had not experienced any urinary tract infections nor any episodes of balano-posthitis. On examination his foreskin was non-retractile but appeared healthy with no evidence of scarring. His mother was insistent that he needed a circumcision.

Introduction

Young boys often present to their primary care physicians with a non-retractile foreskin, which is a particular concern to the parents. The management of this common condition is variable and an accurate diagnosis is required to ensure that young boys are not subjected to an unnecessary procedure. This chapter discusses the natural history of the foreskin and the pathological basis of non-retractile foreskins together with the current treatment recommendations.

History

The key points in the history should ascertain whether the patient has had any urinary tract infections diagnosed or recurrent balano-posthitis. The presentation and symptoms of urinary tract infections in neonates and young males can be non-specific although significant infections are normally diagnosed after investigations in hospital (refer to Chapter 17). The fact that the foreskin is non-retractile at this age is not an indication for circumcision. The ballooning of the prepuce again is not an indication for the procedure. An understanding of the natural history of the foreskin is essential to justify a conservative approach to the management of phimosis.

Examination

The prepuce should be examined to ascertain whether it appears normal or has any evidence of scarring and white patches suggestive of balanitis xerotica obliterans (discussed further on).

Investigations

None are necessary.

Management and discussion

Normal anatomy and development of the foreskin

The foreskin (prepuce) develops from ectoderm, neuroectoderm and mesenchyme to form a double layered fold of skin that envelopes the glans penis. The outer layer is continuous with the penile shaft skin, the inner layer on the other hand is a mucous membrane which lies in direct contact with the glans penis. The foreskin first appears in the foetus at 8 weeks and grows to fully enclose the glans by the 16th week. At this stage the epithelial lining of the inner preputial layer is fused with the epithelium covering the glans penis. Epithelial

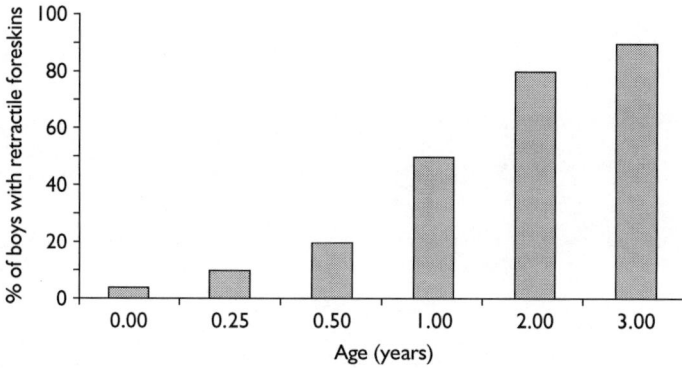

Figure 16.1 The incidence of fully retractile foreskins in early childhood. Adapted from Gairdner (1949).

desquamation, spontaneous erections and penile growth eventually lead to the separation of these two layers of skin.

Seminal work by Gairdner in 1949 provided an insight into the natural history of the release of these two layers of skin. He showed that at birth only 4% of boys had a fully retractile foreskin. The proportion of boys with a fully retractile foreskin increased over time such that by 3 years of age, only 10% of boys still had a 'physiological phimosis' (Figure 16.1). Oster (1968) extended the duration of follow-up and showed that the incidence of phimosis continued to decline with age; he noted that by age 16 years only 1% of boys still had non-retractile foreskins. This process of retractility is spontaneous and does not require manipulation.

Examination of the foreskin

By definition, a phimosis describes the inability to retract the foreskin behind the glans penis. As has just been discussed, this is a normal developmental process during early childhood. A physiological phimosis arises as a result of persistent preputial adhesions and is distinct from a pathological phimosis, where the inability to retract the foreskin is secondary to scarring related to an underlying pathological process such as balanitis xerotica obliterans. When examining the normal childhood foreskin, gentle partial retraction of a non-retractile prepuce shows a characterisitic 'flowering' whereby the inner preputial layer comes into view (Figure 16.2). In a true pathological phimosis there is no flowering and there is evidence of scarring of the prepuce (Figure 16.3).

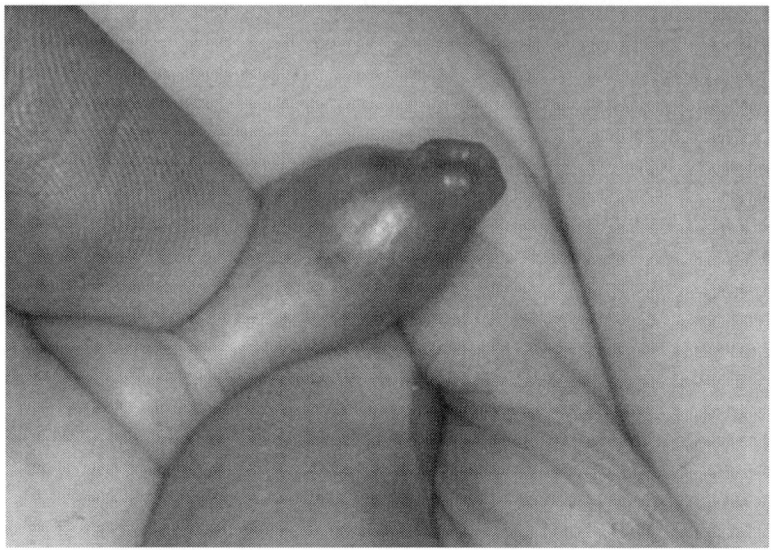

Figure 16.2 Characteristic 'flowering' indicating a physiological phimosis.

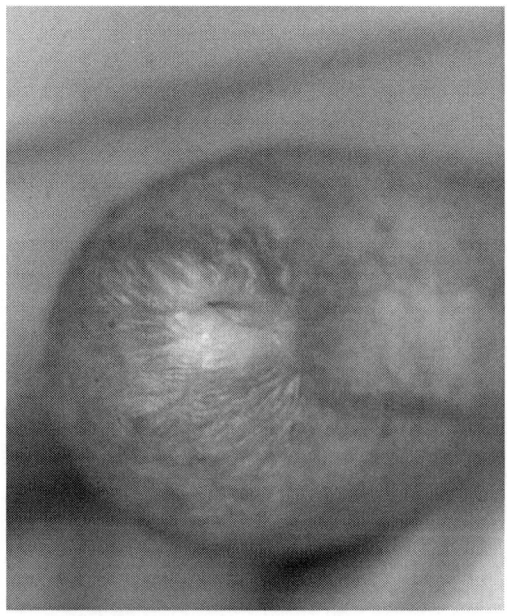

Figure 16.3 True pathological phimosis secondary to balanitis xerotica obliter-ans (BXO) showing scarring and white patches.

Treatment of phimosis

Conservative management

A significant proportion of children with a physiological phimosis are symptom-free and present to their doctors as a result of parental concern. Some boys, however, are symptomatic and can present with voiding difficulty, pain and ballooning upon micturition.

The current guidelines from the American Academy of Pediatrics (AAP), the British Association of Paediatric Surgery (BAPS) and the European Association of Urology (EAU) suggest that these patients can safely be managed conservatively with parental reassurance and advice on bathing and maintaining proper foreskin hygiene.

In patients in whom the foreskin is slow to release, the administration of topical steroid (e.g. 0.1% triamcinolone) twice daily for 6–8 weeks has been shown to accelerate the release of a physiological phimosis in 70–80% of boys. The use of topical steroids has been shown to have no significant side effects or systemic toxicity. There is no evidence to suggest that a physiological phimosis will progress to a pathological one at any stage.

Surgical management of phimosis

The AAP, BAPS and EAU currently recommend surgery in the following circumstances.

- **Balanitis xerotica obliterans (BXO)**
  Balanitis xerotica obliterans is a chronic skin condition of unknown aetiology and is also known as lichen sclerosis et atrophicus. It affects the glans penis, foreskin and occasionally the navicular fossa of the urethra. BXO affects 1.5% of boys and usually presents after the age of 5 years with voiding symptoms and a tight phimosis. Physical examination reveals a thickened white scarred prepuce with no pouting upon retraction (Figure 16.3). It has been suggested controversially that BXO may have an association with the development of penile cancer in adults, though there is no evidence to suggest that this is also the case in children.
- **Recurrent balanoposthitis**
  Balanoposthitis decribes inflammation of the foreskin and glans penis. This condition affects 1% of boys and presents with an erthythematous and oedematous phimosis, often with associated discharge and bleeding. The

most common causative pathogens are *E. coli* and *Proteus*. Initial management comprises bathing, topical steroids and oral antibiotics.

The EAU and BAPS recommend surgery for recurrent balanoposthitis, especially if associated with scarring. These surgical options include circumcision and preputioplasty.

- **Recurrent urinary tract infections in boys with abnormal urinary tracts**
  Numerous studies have demonstrated that uncircumcised boys have a 3–7-fold increased risk of developing urinary tract infections compared to circumcised boys. However, it has also been shown that 111 neonatal circumcisions need to be performed to prevent one UTI. As such, the BAPS and the EAU currently recommend circumcision only in high-risk patients such as those with abnormal urinary tracts (e.g. vesico-ureteric reflux) and those with recurrent UTIs.

Circumcision for non-medical indications

Neonatal, religious or ritual circumcision is still routinely practised throughout the world. Circumcision is the most commonly performed surgical procedure in the USA, with 61% of neonates undergoing surgery. The two main religions whereby circumcision is routinely practised are Islam and Judaism.

Circumcision and prevention of squamous cell carcinoma and sexually transmitted diseases

Squamous cell carcinomas of the penis are extremely rare, affecting 1 in 100,000 men in the USA. Although penile cancer is recognised as being more common in uncircumcised men, there is very little conclusive evidence that routine neonatal circumcision protects against the development of penile cancer as an adult. Acknowledged risk factors for the development of penile cancer are phimosis, poor hygiene, multiple sexual partners, smoking and human papilloma virus infection. The current consensus of the AAP, BAPS and the EAU is that circumcision should not be recommended as a prevention strategy for penile cancer.

Circumcision is believed to have a protective effect against the development of sexually transmitted diseases such as syphilis and human papilloma virus. A study published in the *New England Journal of Medicine* in 2002 reported that male circumcision was associated with a reduced risk of penile HPV infection and, in the case of men with a history of multiple sexual partners, a reduced risk of cervical cancer in their current female partners. The BAPS state that the current evidence is inadequate to recommend routine male circumcision as a preventive measure against cervical cancer.

Two recently published randomised controlled trials have shown that elective adult male circumcisions in endemic areas in Africa reduce the incidence of HIV infection by over 50%. The mucous membrane of the inner preputial skin of the uncircumcised penis is rich in dendritic cells and it is believed that these cells act as target receptors for HIV virus. It must be remembered that transmission of sexually transmitted diseases is multi-factorial and that at present there is no data to suggest that non-therapeutic neonatal circumcision would impact upon the incidence of these diseases.

Surgical technique of circumcision

Elective circumcision for medical reasons should be performed under a general anaesthetic using the sleeve technique. The BAPS do not recommend performing an elective circumcision before the age of one and even then only with the help of an experienced paediatric anaesthetist. The two most commonly performed surgical techniques are described below.

Sleeve technique for circumcision

1. Prior to surgery the patient receives a general anaesthetic with a caudal anaesthetic block.
2. The operative field is prepared with chlorhexadine solution. If possible the foreskin is retracted and any preputial adhesions released. The urethral meatus is inspected to ensure there is no co-existing hypospadius.
3. A free hand scalpel incision is made on the inner preputial skin below the coronal sulcus. The frenulum is also divided if required.
4. The foreskin is replaced and a further free hand scalpel incision is made on the outer skin of the foreskin in line with the coronal sulcus.
5. The section of foreskin between the two incisions is then excised with scissors.
6. Haemostasis is secured using bipolar diathermy. Diathermy must be used with caution near the urethra.
7. The skin edges are sutured using interrupted 5.0 or 4.0 vicryl rapide.

Plastibell circumcision

Most neonatal circumcisions are performed using the Plastibell technique. The BAPS, EAU and the AAP all recommend that this surgery is perfomed using adequate local anaesthesia, which can be administered via a dorsal penile nerve block, a ring block or topical EMLA cream.

1. Once anaesthetised a specially designed plastic bell is placed between the glans penis and the foreskin; an initial dorsal slit may be required to permit this.
2. The foreskin is then pulled slightly forward and a suture looped and tied tightly around the outer layer of the foreskin level with a groove in the plastic bell.
3. The thread cuts off the blood supply to the foreskin which withers and drops off, taking the Plastibell with it. It is usual to remove the excess fore-skin after the knot is tied.

Complications of surgery

The incidence of post-operative complications following circumcision varies between 0.034% and 7.4%. Hospital-based surgery results in lower compli-cation rates when compared with community-based procedures. The most common early complications include oozing of blood, prolonged discomfort, infection needing antibiotics and haemorrhage (2%). Later complications include the removal of too much or too little skin, glanular adhesions, cosmeti-cally poor appearance (4%), inclusion cysts, skin bridging, denuding of the penis, abnormal rotation or chordee of the penis, altered sensation and meatal stenosis (the latter in up to 10%). Major complications such as partial penile amputation and formation of urethra-cutaneous fistula are rare. Most of these complications are preventable with the application of good surgical technique and a modicum of care. The estimated death rate following infant circumcision is 1 in 500,000.

Contraindications for surgery

Elective circumcision is contraindicated in the presence of co-existing con-genital penile anomalies such as a hypospadias. In these circumstances the foreskin may need to be utilised during any future reconstructive surgery. Neonatal circumcision should be avoided in the presence of a hydrocoele or hernia as this increases the risk of developing a post-operative buried penis. Other contraindications include coagulopathies and acute local infections.

Legal aspects of non-medical circumcision

Circumcision for non-medical indications is still controversial. There has been debate as to whether circumcision is a prerequisite in a neonate to be accepted into the Jewish religion and some individuals have taken the option of undergoing procedures to be uncircumcised.

The International Convention on the Rights of the Child states in Article 8 that 'States Parties undertake to respect the right of the child to preserve his or her identity'. Furthermore, Article 14 supports the parents' right to bring up their child according to established ritual or religious practices. Therefore, in the context of religious circumcision in Muslim and Jewish communities, the parents have a right to consent to circumcision, as a failure to do so would be to the detriment of the child's welfare and possible exclusion from their community. However, opponents of ritual or non-medical circumcision argue that the procedure is not medically indicated as the child is not suffering from an illness which would result in disability or death if the treatment was not undertaken. Therefore these bodies propose that circumcision should be postponed until the child has the capacity to make an informed decision. In a survey of American men who were circumcised as neonates, only 0.3% indicated that they would have undergone the procedure in later life if given the option. Therefore parents should be counselled regarding neonatal circumcision and need to be aware that they should act in accordance with what the child may wish for themselves.

Key points

- Non-retractile foreskins are normal in early childhood. Fifty per cent of 1-year-olds have a physiological phimosis, the incidence of which decreases to 10% at 3 years and 1% at 16 years of age.
- A short course (6–8 weeks) of topical corticosteroids can help to release a physiological phimosis.

- A pathologic phimosis arises as a result of scarring related to an underlying pathology (e.g. BXO). A pathological phimosis is an absolute indication for circumcision.
- Relative indications for circumcision include recurrent balanoposthitis and recurrent UTIs in the presence of an abnormal urinary tract.
- There is insufficient evidence to justify routine neonatal circumcision on non-medical grounds.

Further reading and bibliography

Gairdner, D. (1949) The fate of the foreskin, a study of circumcision. *Br. Med. J.*, **2**, 1433–7.

Oster, J. (1968) Further fate of the foreskin. Incidence of preputial adhesions, phimosis, and smegma among Danish schoolboys. *Arch. Dis. Child.*, **43**, 200–3.

Riedmiller, H., Androulakakis, P., Beurton, D., Kocvara, R. and Gerharz, E. (2001) European Association of Urology. EAU guidelines on paediatric urology. *Eur Urol.*, **40**, 589–99.

Statement from the British Association of Paediatric Urologists on behalf of the British Association of Paediatric Surgeons and The Association of Paediatric Anaesthetists. Management of Foreskin Conditions (2008) http://www.baps.org.uk/documents/circumcision2007.pdf; accessed June 2008.

CHAPTER 17

Urinary tract infection in children

Shekhar Marathe, Jas Kalsi and Miranda Ruston

Case history

A 5-month-old female child presents to the GP with her mother. The mother states that her daughter has had fever for two days and 3–4 episodes of vomiting on the first day of illness, and additionally has loose stools. The GP's initial clinical impression was gastroenteritis. She was sent home as the vomiting had settled.

She returns to the practice now because of persistent fever. Vomiting and diarrhoea have resolved. Her mother notes that her urine seems 'strong' and that she is not as playful as usual. She has no cough or rash. She is reviewed again by the GP and a cloudy urine specimen is obtained which is positive for leukocyte esterase and nitrite tests. This is sent for culture.

Introduction

Urinary tract infections (UTIs) are a common and potentially serious condition in young children. During childhood, UTI occurs in about 3–5% of girls and 1% of boys. Most of the UTIs in boys occur in the first year of life. After 2 years of age, UTI in females exceeds that in males by a factor of 10:1. Uncircumcised males less than one year old are more likely to be affected than circumcised males (NICE, 2008). The prevalence of UTI in a febrile child 2–24 months of age, without other source of infection, is 5%.

Why is this condition important?

- It is a common disease in children
- Collecting a urine sample may not be easy
- It is difficult to recognise symptoms and signs
- Children will carry the burden of complications into adult life

Classification

UTIs are divided into two major groups:

1. Those involving the upper urinary tract (pyelonephritis)
2. Those involving the lower urinary tract (cystitis)

Lower tract disease usually does not cause fever, and does not result in renal damage. However, upper tract disease commonly presents with fever, abdominal/flank pain, and in younger children and infants may present with the non-specific symptoms such as poor feeding, irritability, failure to thrive or vomiting and diarrhoea. Even one episode of pyelonephritis can result in significant renal scarring.

Additionally it is important to note several definitions.

1. Recurrent UTI is defined as (over a 1-year period or less):
   - three or more episodes of UTI with cystitis (lower urinary tract infection)
   - two or more episodes of UTI with acute pyelonephritis (upper urinary tract infection)
   - one episode of UTI with acute pyelonephritis plus one or more episodes of UTI with cystitis
2. Atypical UTI includes those associated with any of the following:
   - Seriously ill
   - Infection with non-*E. coli* organisms
   - Septicaemia
   - Raised creatinine
   - Failure to respond to appropriate antibiotics within 48 hours
   - Poor urine flow
   - Abdominal or bladder mass

History

The clinical presentation of UTI varies with the age of the child. Children in their first year may present with vomiting, lethargy, irritability or fever. In those over 6 years and adolescents, presentation may be with dysuria, urgency or frequency, and they may have associated fever, chills, flank pain or hae-maturia. Children 2–6 years of age can present with similar features or may have more non-specific signs, such as abdominal pain, altered voiding pattern, changes to continence, decreased appetite or general malaise.

From infancy to 2 years of age, fever alone is the most common pres-entation of UTI. There may be associated vomiting, constipation, diarrhoea, poor feeding or irritability, but in clinical practice these features do not help in distinguishing UTI from other causes of fever. Vomiting and diarrhoea are at times wrongly diagnosed as symptoms of gastroenteritis. A history of foul-smelling urine or crying on voiding is helpful when present, but absence of these complaints does not rule out UTI. In this age group, UTI should also be considered in the differential diagnosis of failure to attain milestones. Impor-tantly, the possibility of UTI should be considered in any febrile child under 24 months of age. Moreover, girls under 2 years of age and boys under 6 months of age are at highest risk.

Examination

The priority in the physical examination of the child with suspected UTI is to assess the overall degree of illness severity of the child, including hydration status and level of alertness. Vital signs and weight must be recorded. The abdomen should be examined for any masses or tenderness, including renal angle tenderness. Genitalia should be examined for signs of trauma, urethral discharge or phimosis (although particularly < 1 year of age phimosis should be considered normal). The spine should be inspected for skin dimples/pits and also palpated to assess the vertebrae in order to exclude the presence of an underlying spinal cord/vertebral abnormality (e.g. spina bifida). In selected cases, rectal examination (assessing anal sensation, tone and reflexes) may provide further information to exclude a neurologic abnormality.

Urine collection methods

The diagnosis of UTI requires culture of a properly collected urine specimen. In children less than 2 years of age, a properly collected urine specimen may require an invasive procedure: either the gold standard technique of suprapubic aspiration (under ultrasound guidance) or transurethral catheterisation – these techniques are impractical in primary care and should only be performed in the hospital setting.

An alternative in this age group is a bag specimen of urine (BSU), in which a plastic bag, which has a sticky strip, is attached over the baby's/infant's genital area after cleaning very well with soap and water (for boys, the entire penis can go in the bag; for girls the bag goes over the labia). However, BSUs can have false positive rates of up to 50–60% due to contamination by skin commensals. Another option is to use urine collection pads, which are placed inside the nappy and checked every 10 minutes until wet (but not soiled) and then the urine is aspirated with a syringe (gauze or sanitary pads should not be used).

Another method that can be used in this age group and in those over 2 years of age, who cannot void on command, is to obtain a clean catch urine specimen. A clean catch urine sample means that the urethral meatus should be clean, and if possible urine collected should be from the middle of the stream. For girls, cleaning involves separating the labia and cleaning the area. For circumcised boys, the glans of the penis should be cleaned. For uncircumcised boys the foreskin is gently retracted (where possible) prior to cleaning. After cleaning, the child voids, with the parent 'catching' the urine in a clean specimen container after the first few drops are passed. In those who can void on command, the child can void over the toilet and a clean catch mid-stream voided urine specimen may be easily obtained. In girls it is easy to have the child sit facing backwards on the toilet seat, so the carer/parent can easily catch the urine stream from behind the child. Although obtaining clean catch samples can be time consuming and messy, this technique has a high sensitivity and specificity for diagnosing UTIs.

Investigations

Urinalysis

Urinalysis is helpful in evaluating the likelihood of UTI, but cannot definitively exclude it. The most informative components are the leucocyte esterase test, nitrite test and microscopy. Sensitivity is markedly improved when all three are used, although specificity is lower. A positive leucocyte esterase or positive nitrite test is suggestive of UTI, as are more than 5 WBC per HPF (high power field) of a spun urine specimen, or bacteria present on a gram stain of an unspun urine.

Urine culture results are expressed quantitatively, indicating the colony-forming units (CFU or colony count) of bacterial growth. The significance of a positive culture depends upon the method of specimen collection and the number of colonies of a single organism. A colony count of greater than or equal to 100,000 (10^5) is considered significant on properly obtained urine specimens. However, lesser colony counts may also be significant. A specimen obtained by suprapubic aspiration should be sterile, so any growth of gram negative bacteria or any more than a few thousand gram positive cocci is considered a positive culture.

The most common causative agents of UTI are gram negative colonic bacteria, with *Escherichia coli* (*E. coli*) as the commonest cause, followed by *Klebsiella*, *Proteus* and *Enterobacter* species. Gram positive organisms include *Staphylococcus* species and *Enterococcus* species.

Radiological investigations

Recent NICE guidelines have been issued to allow rational and cost-effective radiological investigations to be requested (Table 17.1). Importantly, these are generally requested in secondary care, but clearly, GPs should have a working understanding of them, for obvious reasons. As can be observed, investigations are dependent on whether the UTI resolves in 48 hours, is an atypical UTI or

Table 17.1 Guidelines for imaging in paediatric UTI (adapted from NICE guidelines 2007).

UTI	Age	USS in acute infection	USS in 6/52	DMSA in 4–6/12	MCUG*
Responds well < 48 h	< 6 months		Yes		
Responds well < 48 h	6 months–3 years				
Responds well < 48 h	> 3 years				
Atypical UTI	< 6 months	Yes		Yes	Yes
Atypical UTI	6 months–3 years	Yes		Yes	Consider
Atypical UTI	> 3 years	Yes			
Recurrent UTI	< 6 months	Yes		Yes	Yes
Recurrent UTI	6 months–3 years		Yes	Yes	Consider
Recurrent UTI	> 3 years		Yes	Yes	

USS – ultrasound renal tract; DMSA – dimercaptosuccinic acid renogram; MCUG – micturating cystourethrogram
*Some centres may prefer MAG3 (mercaptoacetyltriglycine) renogram with indirect cystogram in cases suspected to have vesicoureteric reflux

is a recurrent UTI. In all children, except those less than 6 months, with a UTI that resolves within 48 hours, no further investigations are merited. In those less than 6 months, a renal tract ultrasound is performed after 6 weeks. Atypical UTIs and recurrent UTIs generally require further radiological assessment to establish a possible cause (Table 17.1).

Management and discussion

The various treatment modalities are also based on recommendations based on NICE guidelines. It is convenient to divide patients into three groups for acute management:

1. Infants younger than 3 months – refer urgently to paediatric specialist unit for parenteral antibiotics.
2. Infants and children 3 months or older with pyelonephritis – refer urgently to a paediatric specialist unit. Immediate treatment with oral antibiotics for 7–10 days is commenced. Oral antibiotics such as cephalosporin or co-amoxiclav are recommended, as these have the advantage of low resistance. If the child cannot tolerate oral antibiotics, intravenous (IV) antibiotic agents such as cefotaxime or ceftriaxone for 2–4 days are considered. This can be later changed to an oral dose if possible. Treatment continues for 10–14 days.
3. Infants and children 3 months or older with cystitis – the general practitioner may commence with oral antibiotics for 3 days. Trimethoprim, cephalosporin, nitrofurantoin or amoxicillin are recommended. Local guidelines can differ from place to place. Ask the child/infant to be brought back for reassessment if child is still unwell after 24 hours. Do remember to chase the urine culture result or send a fresh sample

Choice of antibiotic

The initial choice of antimicrobials is guided by the route of administration, known uropathogens and the baseline renal function of the child. It is adjusted based on clinical response and results of culture and sensitivity testing. Initial oral therapy may be with trimethoprim or with a cephalosporin (e.g. cephalexin). The oral drug nitrofurantoin is excreted in the urine, but it does not reach good concentrations in blood or tissues. It therefore has little value in treating febrile UTIs in infants/children.

Parenteral therapy may be with a cephalosporin (e.g. ceftriaxone, cefotaxime) or ampicillin/co-amoxiclav. An aminoglycoside should be used with caution in renal impairment.

As regards antibiotic prophylaxis, this should not be considered in children presenting with their first UTI. Additionally there is no place for prophylaxis in asymptomatic bacteriuria. However, it can be started in those with recurrent UTIs.

Vesico-ureteric reflux

Vesico-ureteric reflux (VUR) is present in 30–50 % of children with UTI, and these patients are at increased risk of renal damage from UTIs. Children with recurrent or atypical UTIs need to be investigated with renal ultrasound and MCUG. If studies are delayed until after completion of 7–14 days of antibiotic therapy, the child should remain on antimicrobial prophylaxis until the studies are completed. Drugs of choice include trimethoprim and nitrofurantoin, in prophylactic doses. The child with VUR needs long-term follow-up with antibiotic prophylaxis, periodic monitoring of urine cultures, repeat imaging of the urinary tract, and possible surgical intervention (for persistent VUR or recurrent UTIs despite prophylaxis). DMSA scanning is helpful in determining the presence of renal scarring in children with VUR and the degree of renal impairment.

Prognosis

Prognosis after UTI in childhood depends on:

1. Whether the infection was limited to the upper tract or involved the lower tract
2. The presence of VUR
3. The presence of other urinary tract anomalies

Uncomplicated infections without associated obstruction respond well to antibiotic therapy. However, one third of these children may present with recurrence of UTI within the first year after acute infection. In such cases, maintaining a record of follow-up urine cultures is essential. Whilst pyelonephritis and renal scarring can occur in the absence of VUR, the severity of renal scarring often correlates with the degree of reflux. The natural history of low-grade reflux is toward spontaneous resolution, whereas high-grade reflux is less likely to resolve without surgery. The combination of repeated infections and VUR puts children at risk for renal scarring, which may progress to end stage renal disease. However, renal damage can occur before VUR is diagnosed. Early diagnosis and treatment of UTI and VUR is therefore required to reduce the incidence of these long-term complications.

Key points

- Maintain a high index of suspicion for the diagnosis of childhood UTIs.
- Spend time in obtaining an adequate urine specimen for culture.
- Promptly commence empiric antibiotic and change as necessary (depending on sensitivities).
- Appropriate imaging is essential.
- Identify atypical/recurrent cases and arrange further referral.

Further reading and bibliography

NICE (2008) Clinical Guideline 54: Urinary Tract Infection in Children. http://www. nice.org.uk/; accessed June 2008.

Rickwood, A. M. K. (2002) Urinary infection. In: *Essentials of Paediatric Urology* (eds. D. F. M. Thomas, A. M. K. Rickwood and P. G. Duffy), pp. 35–43. Martin Dunitz Ltd, London.

Thomas, D. F. M. (2002) Vesico-ureteric reflux. In: *Essentials of Paediatric Urology* (eds. D. F. M. Thomas, A. M. K. Rickwood and P. G. Duffy), pp. 45–55. Martin Dunitz Ltd, London.

CHAPTER 18

Urinary incontinence in children

*Dawit Worku, Erdinc Havutcu, Jay Khastgir, George Fowlis
and Rim El-Rifai*

Case history

A 6-year-old girl was brought to her GP because of nocturnal bed wetting. She had never previously been dry during the night and was a 'deep
sleeper'. She became dry during the day at the age of 2.5 years. There
were no other urological problems and development was normal. There
were no signs of behavioural or emotional symptoms. The paediatric
examination was normal. She was treated with an alarm and became dry
within a few weeks without nocturia. This is a typical scenario for a child
with primary monosymptomatic nocturnal enuresis.

Introduction

Incontinence refers to any involuntary loss of urine at a socially unacceptable place and time by a child aged 5 years or more whose general cognitive
and neurological development indicates that bladder control should have been
achieved. It is very common during childhood and is in more than 95% of cases
functional (i.e. not caused by disease, injury or congenital malformation) rather
than organic in aetiology. This said, organic causes must be excluded to prevent
irreversible deterioration in renal function. The organic causes can be either
structural (e.g. ectopic ureter or epispadias) or neurogenic (e.g. spina bifida).

Urinary incontinence in children is subdivided into night-time/nocturnal
(most common) and daytime incontinence. Additionally, primary incontinence refers to the group in which there has never been a prolonged dry spell,
whereas in secondary incontinence the child has previously been dry for at
least 6 months.

The aetiology of childhood incontinence is multifactorial. Genetic factors are important in the aetiology of nocturnal enuresis, while environmental factors may exert a modulatory effect. Some children have been found to have nocturnal polyuria secondary to relative night-time deficiency of the antidiuretic hormone vasopressin. Furthermore, given the prominent role of detrusor (bladder muscle) overactivity (instability) in the pathogenesis of daytime incontinence, and the overlap between the groups of bedwetting and day-wetting children, it is believed that it may play a crucial role in the pathogenesis of a subgroup of enuretic children. In addition, it is believed that the 'deep sleep' of enuretic children may at least play a permissive role in the pathogenesis of enuresis, since both bladder distension and detrusor contractions are strong arousal stimuli. Finally, epidemiological studies have shown that 20–30% of all nocturnal enuretic children show clinically relevant behavioural problems (e.g. withdrawal, physical complaints, anxiousness/depression, social problems and internalising behaviour) at a 2–4 times higher rate than non-wetting children.

Nocturnal incontinence

Night-time incontinence or nocturnal enuresis denotes bedwetting or passing urine in bed while asleep, in a child who has passed his or her fifth birthday. Nocturnal enuresis is a common problem among children and adolescents. If a frequency of at least one 'wet night' per month is used as the definition, the prevalence may be as high as 10% among 6-year-olds, 5% among 10-year-olds, and 0.5–1.0% among teenagers and young adults. Nocturnal enuresis may be primary (lifelong) or (secondary where there has been a dry interval of at least six months). Nocturnal enuresis may be the sole symptom, in which case it may be called monosymptomatic nocturnal enuresis. If it is associated with other urinary symptoms, such as severe urgency and frequency (i.e. symptoms of an overactive/unstable bladder), the condition is sometimes referred to as polysymptomatic nocturnal enuresis. A functional (rather than organic) cause can be assumed in monosymptomatic nocturnal enuresis.

Daytime incontinence

Approximately 5% of 7-year-olds suffer from daytime urinary incontinence. The decreasing prevalence with increasing age of the child, as seen in nocturnal enuresis, is less clear here, and in adulthood the prevalence rises again, especially among women. Most cases of daytime incontinence are considered to be functional. Functional day-wetting is incontinence not caused by disease, injury or congenital malformation.

The main syndromes that constitute functional urinary incontinence include urge incontinence, voiding postponement, dysfunctional voiding, stress incontinence, giggle incontinence and detrusor underactivity.

- Urge incontinence due to an overactive bladder is urinary incontinence in a child who experiences urgency symptoms but does not regularly postpone micturition or exhibit holding manoeuvres. The child voids frequently and the voided volumes are typically small.
- Voiding postponement is a term used in those children who habitually postpone micturition, using various holding manoeuvres such as crossing their legs, often until it is too late, and incontinence is the result.
- Dysfunctional voiding denotes the tendency towards intermittent or continuous sphincter contractions during bladder emptying, commonly resulting in residual urine and possibly urinary tract infections.
- Stress incontinence is a very rare condition in the neurologically intact child, which occurs on exertion and is caused by an underactive (or damaged) sphincter.
- Giggle incontinence is the peculiar and uncommon condition where laughter, specifically, triggers apparently complete bladder emptying.
- Detrusor underactivity (or 'lazy bladder') is defined as the non-neurogenic inability of the detrusor to completely empty the bladder, forcing the child to strain with the abdominal musculature or apply manual suprapubic pressure during micturition, often resulting in incontinence due to bladder overfilling.

Organic urinary incontinence in children is extremely rare and can be due to structural, iatrogenic or neurogenic causes. This requires referral to a specialist paediatric urologist.

History

The importance of a good case history, even in seemingly uncomplicated cases, such as monosymptomatic nocturnal enuresis, can not be overstated.

The history of the enuretic child should initially include questions regarding the type of enuresis, i.e. primary or secondary enuresis, nocturnal or both day- and nighttime incontinence, and monosymptomatic or non-monosymptomatic/polysymptomatic enuresis. This is important because those children with either primary, both day- and night-time, or polysymptomatic urinary incontinence are much more likely to have significant underlying abnormalities.

The severity of the incontinence should be assessed as dry, damp or soaking and the frequency of wetting documented. Associated lower urinary tract symptoms including frequency, urgency +/– incontinence and any symptoms or history of urinary tract infection should be enquired after. General fluid input and excessive thirst may be relevant. Bowel habit and particularly a predilection to constipation should be noted. Children with nocturnal enuresis are frequently deep sleepers and difficult to rouse and subsequently communicate with. This should be documented, as it may reflect on the likely response to alarm treatment. It is also interesting to know whether the disorder runs in the family, although this will not affect treatment. Some brief questions should also be asked about the general health and development of the child. It is important to find out whether the child regards the enuresis as a serious problem and how much it affects his or her life. Possible concomitant behavioural issues may need to be addressed, but a detailed psychiatric evaluation is only needed if the child exhibits overt behavioural or emotional symptoms.

Examination

All children who present with incontinence should undergo a standard physical examination at least once. The physical examination should include height, weight, head circumference, inspection of the genitalia, inspection and palpation of the spine (e.g. looking for evidence of spina bifida) and simple neurological examination (leg reflexes, Babiniski's sign). A rectal examination may be indicated if constipation is suspected. Even at this early stage a simple voiding chart completed by the patient is an invaluable aid when looking for signs of bladder dysfunction or excessive or reduced fluid intake.

Investigations

A thorough clinical history and examination, supported by a voiding chart and a simple urinalysis, should be enough in most instances. Urinalysis is particularly important in children with secondary enuresis, in whom excessive thirst, general malaise or weight loss may indicate diabetes (mellitus or insipidus) or kidney disease. Blood tests or other invasive investigations are not usually needed. Children with enuresis who fail to respond to conventional treatments or those associated with recurrent UTIs should receive the attention of a paediatric specialist.

Specialist investigation may include uroflowmetry and residual urine measurement. This can exclude outflow obstruction and confirm post-void bladder emptying. Ultrasound of the renal tract is not usually required unless there is a history of urine infections – to screen for anatomical abnormalities and renal atrophy/scarring. The use of intravenous urography (IVU) is virtually obsolete nowadays, except in cases of suspected ectopic ureter. In cases of enuresis for a neuropathic cause, cystography may be performed to exclude vesico-ureteric reflux.

Management and discussion

Monosymptomatic nocturnal enuresis

Treatment is indicated when the bedwetting threatens to become a social or psychological problem for the child, starting from the age of 5 years. Simple measures are employed as first line. Information should be given regarding fluid intake (extra fluid in the morning and at lunchtime and avoiding drinking large volumes before bedtime) and regular voiding habits (approximately six voids per day). Ineffective treatment, including punishment, fluid restriction and waking, should be discontinued. Star charts are an effective and simple way of managing nocturnal enuresis. Wet and dry nights are registered on a sheet, rewarding children for dry nights. Usually a period of four weeks is sufficient, but star charts can be used for longer if improvements are seen. Treating constipation with dietary advice and laxatives as necessary is also important.

If simple methods fail, the second line therapy includes the enuresis alarm or desmopressin treatment. The alarm is fitted under the bed sheet and if this becomes wet an electric circuit is completed and the alarm sounds. The child is then encouraged by a parent to void in the toilet. The alarm is potentially curative but demands motivation and commitment by the child and parents. Treatment should be consistent (no weekend interruptions), and continued until 14 consecutive dry nights have been achieved within a maximum of 16 weeks. Alarm treatment can be combined with other behavioural techniques such as 'arousal training'.

If desmopressin is chosen, parents need to be informed about the risk of water intoxication if the drug is combined with excessive fluid intake. Desmopressin is given orally (0.2–0.4 mg) or intranasally (20–40 µg) at bedtime; the doses should be titrated individually. Effects should be evident within a maximum of four weeks. If the child does not respond within this time treatment should be stopped. If it is effective, it can be given at the lowest dose necessary in 12-week blocks, followed by a withdrawal for a week. In the case of relapse, new 'blocks' of up to 12 weeks can be started again.

If both enuresis alarms and desmopressin are ineffective, then anticholinergic medications, possibly in combination with first and second line therapies, may be considered. In specialist units there is still a place for imipramine treatment of therapy-resistant enuresis. Finally, in therapy-resistant cases, detailed urological and child psychiatric assessment, inpatient and day-case treatment may be considered. Subgroups such as those with secondary nocturnal enuresis have a higher rate of co-morbid psychiatric disorders which need to be addressed.

Daytime incontinence

The initial management of daytime incontinence is similar to that of mono-symptomatic nocturnal enuresis, namely regular voiding habits (approximately six times per day) and adjustment of fluid intake. Children are asked to register any signs of urge and go to the toilet immediately and to refrain from using holding manoeuvres. Charts may also be used; each voiding is registered, with different signs for wet (e.g. 'clouds') or dry (e.g. 'flags'). Digital wrist alarm watches can act as useful reminders in older children. Regular follow-up and encouragement are recommended.

The second-line treatment of bladder overactivity is anticholinergic medication (oxybutynin, tolterodine), provided that there is no residual urine. If one anticholinergic is ineffective or not tolerated (dry mouth and constipation are the commonest side effects) switching from one anticholinergic to another is recommended. Bladder training with charts should continue whilst on medication to record and reward success. Long-term antibiotic prophylaxis may be needed in children with overactive bladder and proven concomitant urinary tract infections, whilst the bladder disturbance is treated. If co-morbid behavioural and emotional symptoms are present, counselling and psychotherapy and other child psychiatric interventions might be indicated.

Dysfunctional voiding is associated with a high risk of UTIs, faecal soiling and constipation, requiring further therapy. In addition to providing information and regulation of voiding and drinking habits, the most effective form of treatment is biofeedback training. A visual biofeedback with uroflow can be employed. Relaxation techniques may be added. Residual urine should be checked after each void. In most cases, coordination can be achieved on an outpatient basis.

Genuine stress incontinence is extremely rare in children. If genuine stress incontinence is suspected in a child, a specialist referral for urodynamics is appropriate.

In giggle incontinence, regulation of voiding and drinking habits should be encouraged. The main lines of treatment are either pharmacological (stimulant medication at a dose higher than in the treatment of ADHD) or cognitive-behavioural.

Finally, children with bladder underactivity need to be evaluated with a voiding chart and with repeated uroflow measurements and assessment of residual urine. Ultrasound of the kidneys and urinary tracts should also be performed to exclude upper tract dilation and risk of permanent renal damage. Regular toileting, every 2 hours with time to allow complete bladder emptying on each occasion, is recommended. Constipation, if present, should be treated, and some children may need antibiotic prophylaxis until residual urine has disappeared.

Summary

Enuresis and particularly nocturnal enuresis is a common problem. The most common cause is functional voiding problems and organic causes are rare. Nevertheless, it is important to exclude organic causes to minimise potential loss of renal function. Treatments initially involve conservative treatments with advice about fluid input and regular voids during the day and treating constipation. If these fail second line treatments may be employed, including pharmaceuticals. In medication-resistant children or in those with an organic or emotional/behavioural cause, specialist care is recommended.

Key points

■ Incontinence refers to any involuntary loss of urine at a socially unacceptable place and time by a child aged 5 years with normal cognitive and neurological development.
■ Nocturnal enuresis represents the commonest form of incontinence in children.
■ Most cases of daytime incontinence can be considered to be functional forms of urinary incontinence.

> - The importance of good case history, even in seemingly uncompli-
>   cated cases of incontinence in children, cannot be overstated.
> - The first line treatment for nocturnal enuresis is enuresis alarm or
>   desmopressin.

Further reading and bibliography

Rickwood, A. M. K. (2002) Urinary incontinence. In: *Essentials of Paediatric Urology* (eds. D. F. M. Thomas, A. M. K. Rickwood and P. G. Duffy), pp. 125–34. Martin Dunitz Ltd, London.

CHAPTER 19

Cryptorchidism

Dawit Worku, Mohamed Hammadeh, Penelope Cox and George Fowlis

Case history

A 6-month-old boy was brought in by a concerned parent because his scrotum appeared empty on his left side. He was otherwise a healthy and playful child. He was reported to have had low birth weight and pre-term delivery. On examination, his left testis was palpated at the level of the external inguinal ring and couldn't be brought down to a dependent position in the scrotum. No anomalies or other findings were noted on further examination.

This is a typical scenario for unilateral cryptorchidism without associated anomalies. The boy was treated with a standard orchidopexy with satisfactory outcome.

Introduction

The word 'cryptorchid' comes from Greek word cryptos, meaning hidden, and orchis, meaning testis, and thus cryptorchidism literally means 'hidden testis'. This term is frequently applied to all forms of undescended testes, including palpable, impalpable and ectopic testis, and generally signifies the presence of an empty scrotum. The word 'cryptorchidism' is almost interchangeable with the term 'undescended testis' except that the latter does not include testes that may be manipulated into the scrotum, e.g. 'retractile testis'.

Overall, 3% of full-terms and 30% of premature newborn boys are born with at least one undescended testis (UDT), making isolated UDT one of the most common congenital anomalies found at birth. Most undescended testis descend spontaneously by the first year of life (about 70% to 77% by 3 months of age), thus reducing the incidence to 1% by 1 year of age. The right side is more commonly affected and 25% of cases are bilateral.

The cause of UDT is multifactorial. Low birth weight and prematurity predispose to the condition, but frequently these testes will descend in early infancy. Testicular descent is under hormonal control and in full-term infants an imbalance in this is the likely aetiology.

Cryptorchid testes are usually classified as either palpable or impalpable. If impalpable, testes may be intra-abdominal or absent (vanishing testes). If palpable, testes may be undescended, ectopic or retractile. Approximately 80% of undescended testes are clinically palpable and 20% are impalpable.

An intra-abdominal testis can be located anywhere along the line between the lower pole of the kidney and the internal inguinal ring, although it is usually found just inside the internal ring. The hallmark of a vanishing or absent testis is blind-ending spermatic vessels that are found just proximal to the internal inguinal ring, and is thought to occur from an intrauterine or prenatal vascular event. An ectopic testis is a condition in which the testis has descended but occupies an abnormal position, usually in the perineum, though they may be found lateral to the scrotum, in the thigh or suprapubic region. Retractile testis may be palpated anywhere along the natural course of the testis, but most are inguinal. Although not truly cryptorchid, a retractile testis withdraws spontaneously out of the scrotum toward the inguinal canal by an active cremasteric reflex, but can easily be brought down into a dependent position within the scrotum and remains there after traction has been released. The cremasteric reflex is usually weak during infancy and most active in boys aged 5 years, hence the common occurrence of retractile testis between the ages of 3 and 7 years.

Cryptorchidism is associated with a number of complications. Impairment of germ cell maturation leading to subfertility or infertility is one such important complication, requiring early surgical repositioning of the testis into the scrotum before the onset of histopathologic changes that increases the risk for subfertility. Changes can be seen on electron microscopy at 1 year, so the optimal age for surgical correction is at 6–18 months, allowing sufficient time for natural descent whilst minimising long-term testis damage. Children born with undescended testes are also at increased risk for testicular malignancy. Approximately 10% of testicular tumours arise from an undescended testis. The relative risk of testicular cancer among boys who undergo orchiopexy before reaching 13 years of age is 2.23, as compared with the general population; for those treated at 13 years of age or older, the relative risk is 5.40. Bringing the testis down does not appear to reduce the incidence of developing cancer significantly in pubertal boys; it does, however, make a tumour more easily palpable.

A patent processus vaginalis is found in more than 90% of patients with an undescended testis. Hence several authors report an incidence of accompanying hernia in more than 65%. Furthermore, although testicular torsion is an uncommon condition, a significant number of such patients are reported to be cryptorchid. The increased susceptibility of the testis is the result of a developmental anatomic abnormality between the testis and its mesentery. A cryptorchid testis lying in the inguinal canal is more vulnerable to trauma than is the normally descended gonad. In addition, an empty scrotum may be a source of considerable anxiety and embarrassment, often causing feelings of physical inferiority and concern about virility.

History

Frequently, the child who presents with undescended testis has no other symptoms. Although some parents are poor historians when it comes to observation of their son's scrotum, the majority will be able to indicate with certainty that the testis has or has not been present in the scrotum at some time since birth. Often the parent will have observed that the testis descends into the scrotum when the boy is taking a warm bath or sleeping, and then retracts into the inguinal canal when stimulated.

Overall, elements of the medical history of children with cryptorchidism should include determination of whether the testis has ever been palpable in scrotum, birth weight, prior inguinal surgery, maternal history including use of gestational steroids, prenatal history (i.e. assisted reproductive technique, maternal hormonal treatment, multiple gestations), history of prematurity if applicable, and family history (i.e. cryptorchidism, hypospadias, intersex, precocious puberty, infertility, consanguinity).

Examination

Careful examination of the boy should take place in a warm consultation room, with warm hands and a warm smile! The abdomen, inguinal region, perineum and scrotum should be examined while the child is relaxed in supine position with knees elevated. In over 85% of patients with cryptorchidism, the testis can be felt at the level of the external inguinal ring or along the course of the inguinal canal.

Once the testis is identified above the level of the scrotum, note should also be made of its size compared with the contralateral testis, as well as its shape and consistency. Furthermore, the examiner should attempt to ascertain whether the testis can be manipulated into the scrotum. This can be achieved by pressing the finger of the examining hand flat against the patient's lower abdomen just above the testis, which should then slowly be brought downwards over the external ring with a sweeping motion in an attempt to manipulate the testis downwards into the scrotum. The fingers of the other hand may assist by grasping the testis when it passes the scrotal neck and directing it into the scrotum as far as possible. This manoeuvre can be repeated while noting the lower-most location in which the testis can be positioned, e.g. low inguinal canal, superficial inguinal pouch, high scrotum, or low scrotum (normal). If the testis cannot be manipulated into the scrotum, further examination of the patient in a standing or sitting position with the legs crossed may assist the testis to descend slightly lower.

Occasionally, optimal examination of particularly hyperactive or unusually 'ticklish' child may be difficult. Boys who are listed for orchidopexy are therefore examined whilst asleep before making an incision to ensure the testis is undescended and requiring surgery rather than retractile and in no need of intervention.

Investigation

In children suspected of having an undescended testis, determination of whether the testis is present on physical examination is critically important as it guides further workup and treatment. Approximately 20% of undescended testes are impalpable. Most impalpable testes are intra-abdominal, the remainder being intracanalicular or absent. Approximately 20% of impalpable testes are absent and 30% are atrophic.

For unilateral undescended testes without hypospadious on clinical examination, no further investigations are required and we thus recommend referral to a urologist once the diagnosis has been clinically confirmed. The ability of radiologic investigations to identify the site of an undescended testis is 44%. Many modalities have been used, including ultrasound, computed tomography, magnetic resonance imaging, testicular angiography and venography. Many of these techniques are invasive, require anaesthesia, are technically difficult to perform, or are associated with a significant rate of false negative results. Therefore in secondary care surgical exploration is undertaken to identify the site of the testis, assess its viability and then bring down or excise as necessary.

The presentation of bilateral undescended testes is very rare in primary care and the workup for bilateral impalpable testes, which occurs in the hospital setting, merits special consideration because it may represent a life-threatening situation if it is associated with either hypospadias or ambiguous genitalia. First intersex (females with adrenal hyperplasia) should be ruled out. The diagnosis of bilateral anorchia should be considered if a male karyotype is confirmed. Endocrinologic evaluation is necessary and may help determine whether one or both testes are present. Childhood is a quiescent phase in testicular activity, and the hCG stimulation test is widely used to evaluate testicular function. The hCG stimulation test can be performed to induce testosterone production if at least one testis is present. However, there may be a false negative response if the Leydig cells are unresponsive to exogenous hCG. If basal gonadotropin levels, FSH in particular, are increased in a prepubescent boy, further endocrine workup is unnecessary because it probably represents bilateral anorchia. If gonadotropin levels are normal in a boy with bilateral impalpable testes, an hCG stimulation test can be performed to further establish the diagnosis.

Management and discussion

The objectives of treatment of a child with an undescended testis include: proper identification of the anatomy, position and viability of the undescended testis; identification of any potential coexisting syndromic abnormalities; placement of the testis in a timely fashion to prevent further testicular impairment in either fertility potential or endocrinologic function; attainment of permanent fixation of the testis with a normal scrotal position that allows for easy palpation and avoid further testicular damage resulting from the treatment.

Definitive treatment of an undescended testis should take place between 6 and 18 months of age. Spontaneous descent occurs in most boys by 3 months of age and uncommonly thereafter. Early intervention should be considered in order to prevent the irreversible testis damage that occurs after 1 year of age. Therefore if the GP clinically diagnoses cryptorchidism the infant should be referred to the urologist between 3 and 6 months of age.

Treatments for undescended testis by the specialist have included medical (hormonal) or surgical, or a combination of the two. Medical treatments of cryptorchidism include exogenous hCG and exogenous GnRH or LHRH. The mechanism of action in both cases increases serum testosterone production by stimulation at different levels of the hypothalamic-pituitary-gonadal cascade. This therapy is based on experimental observation that descent is mediated by androgen and involves testicular synthesis of the active metabolite in high local concentration. hCG stimulates Leydig cells directly to produce testosterone, whereas GnRH stimulates the pituitary to release LH and thereby promote testicular production of testosterone. Successful results have been reported in testes that were retractile; however, in a double blind placebo controlled trial hormonal treatment was ineffective in treating true undescended testes.

Standard (inguinal) orchidopexy is a well-established surgical treatment for a palpable undescended testis. The testis is identified and the cord skeletalised to optimise mobility whilst preserving the important cord structures. The testis is brought into the scrotum and secured in a pouch made in the Dartos muscle of the scrotum. The most significant complication of orchidopexy is testicular atrophy, which is reported in 5% of cases. Dissection of testicular vessels and/or postoperative swelling and inflammation can result in ischemic injury and testicular atrophy. Furthermore, standard orchidopexy is reported to have up to an 8% failure rate, even in the distal undescended testis, and a failure rate of more than 25% for intra-abdominal testes. Other potential complications include damage to the vas, probably under-reported as 2%, ascent of the testis (which would require a second orchidopexy), infection and bleeding. Hence orchidopexy should be performed by urologists who are well versed in the surgical procedure and the management of complications.

The objective of surgical management of the impalpable testis is diagnostic and potentially therapeutic. Initially, it is important to establish the presence of the testis through open inguinal or diagnostic laparoscopic technique. Approximately 20% of impalpable testes are absent, 30% atrophic and about 50% intra-abdominal.

As stated, the two initial surgical approaches to the impalpable testis are the open inguinal and diagnostic laparoscopic techniques. In the open inguinal approach, the groin is explored. If cord structures or testicular remnants are found, they are removed, and the procedure is terminated. If the groin exploration is negative, the incision is extended, and the peritoneum is entered in a search for an intra-abdominal testis. This technique has now been nearly universally superseded by the second approach.

The second surgical approach to the impalpable testis is laparoscopic. Diagnostic laparoscopy, which is a safe procedure in experienced hands, is performed initially. Using a laparoscope placed through the umbilicus, the inguinal rings are examined and the status of the processus vaginalis (patent or non-patent), mesonephric structures and testicular vessels can be easily identified. The presence of blind-ending spermatic vessels confirms an absent testis, allowing termination of the procedure without a groin incision. If vessels and vas deferens exit the internal ring, the inguinal region can be explored. If an intra-abdominal testis is identified, the surgeon can then choose the best surgical approach, either orchidectomy or orchidopexy. The Fowler–Stephens approach may be employed, here the testicular vessels are divided as these are limiting descent. Depending on the site within the abdomen the testis may be left for a few months to establish its collateral blood supply from the artery to the vas. Once this is considered sufficient, the testis is brought down using a laparoscopic assisted orchidopexy.

Key points

- Cryptorchidism is one of the most common congenital anomalies found at birth, affecting upward of 3% of full-term newborns.
- Most cryptorchid testes descend spontaneously by the first year of life, reducing the incidence to 1% by 1 year of age.
- Cryptorchidism is a clinical diagnosis and the use of imaging (e.g. ultrasound) is not necessary due to its low sensitivity.
- The optimal time for initiating treatment for undescended testis is between 6 and 18 months of age, and therefore we recommend referral to a urologist between 3 and 6 months of age.
- After 6 months of age the treatment of an undescended testis is usually surgical.
- The two common surgical techniques are inguinal exploration or laparoscopy.

Further reading and bibliography

Madden, N. P. (2002) Testis, hydrocele and varicocele. In: *Essentials of Paediatric Urology* (eds. D. F. M. Thomas, A. M. K. Rickwood and P. G. Duffy), pp. 189–201. Martin Dunitz Ltd, London.

PART III

Miscellaneous

CHAPTER 20

Urethral catheterisation

Rajesh Kavia, Vinay Kalsi, Christopher Blick, Jayanta Barua and Philippe Grange

The operation of introducing the catheter, if it do not require intrepidity and courage, requires at least peculiar delicacy, a perfect knowledge of the parts, and above all, a humane and steady temper...

John Bell (1810)

Introduction

Male and female urethral catheterisation is commonly performed in clinical practice and is an essential skill for every medical practitioner. The incidence of hospital inpatients having a urethral catheter inserted at some time during admission is of the order of 20% and studies have shown that up to 9% of patients in nursing homes have urinary catheters and 4% of patients living at home, known to a district nursing service, use a long-term indwelling catheter.

Whilst doctors are generally confident with male catheterisation they find catheterising women challenging as this is normally done by the nursing staff in day-to-day practice. In the community, district nurses will manage most with urinary catheters (urethral or suprapubic) and general practitioners (GPs) may only be asked to intervene with the more difficult cases. This chapter outlines the indications for urinary catheterisation and details the techniques for urethral catheterisation, types of catheters used and potential complications encountered.

Indications

Catheters can provide an effective means of draining the bladder for short- or long-term purposes by intermittent or indwelling catheterisation. Catheterisation can be considered short-term for up to 14 days, or long-term for any period of time over 14 days.

Indications for short-term catheterisation include acute urinary retention; monitoring of the urine output; post-surgery; temporary urinary diversion (e.g. patients with pressure sores).

Long-term indwelling catheters may be necessary for patients with bladder outlet obstruction unsuitable for surgery; chronic retention, often as a result of neurological disease or injury (where clean intermittent self catheterisation (CISC) is not possible); conditions resulting in debilitation, paralysis or coma; or intractable incontinence where catheterisation enhances quality of life (only where alternative methods have been inappropriate or exhausted).

Technique of insertion

Patient preparation

As catheterisation is an invasive procedure, the patient should be fully informed and wherever possible the decision to catheterise should be a joint one between the patient, carer (if in a home) and the health professional. Verbal consent at least must be obtained. The procedure involves instrumentation of a potentially sterile tract and an aseptic technique is therefore mandatory. A clean and draped tray should be prepared with the appropriate catheter, a catheter bag, water for injection for inflation of balloon, local anaesthetic gel (10–15 ml of 2% lignocaine hydrochloride gel), cleaning solution and sterile cotton wool and disposable forceps to clean with. Following thorough hand washing and donning sterile gloves, the patient's genital area should be cleaned with sterile water or an antiseptic solution such as 2% chlorhexidine. All efforts need to be made to maintain asepsis and this can effectively be done by double gloving and discarding the top gloves after cleaning, before handling the catheter, or by ensuring that only one hand is used in cleaning whilst the other is used to insert the catheter. The cleaned area is then suitably draped.

Types of catheter and drainage devices

Table 20.1 details the selection of catheter material available according to the indication. Most commonly Foley balloon catheters will be used, the material depending on the duration of its use. Short term catheters are often latex or polyurethane based – these can remain *in situ* for up to two weeks. Longer

Table 20.1 Selection of appropriate catheter material and duration of use.

Duration of catheterisation	Catheter material	Recommended time for catheter change
Intermittent (CISC)	Plastic +/– hydrophilic coating	N/A CISC should be performed according to advice from continence advisor and based on the residual volume of urine obtained per catheterisation
Short-term (up to 14 days)	Latex or polyurethane based	Up to 2 weeks
Medium-term (up to 28 days)	Teflon-coated latex Silver alloy (may also be selected for longer term use and in patients who have a catheter reaction to ordinary catheters)	Up to 4 weeks
Long-term (more than 14 days)	Hydrogel coated latex Silicone-elastomer coated latex All silicone	8–12 weeks

term catheters are silicone-based or PTFE-coated latex; these are suitable for 8–12 weeks. The exact duration for which an individual catheter can be left *in situ* will be provided on the catheter packing.

Standard adult two-way catheter sizes vary form 10 Fr (French) to 18 Fr. Most patients will have a 12 or 14 Fr catheter inserted. One should choose the smallest catheter possible to allow adequate drainage, as urethral secretions drain more easily around smaller catheters. Drainage of these secretions reduces the risk of significant urethral inflammatory response. The standard male catheter length is 41–45 cm and is appropriate for use in both sexes; however, the shorter female catheter of approximately 25 cm may be more comfortable and discrete for some patients. Female length catheters should never be used in men as inflation of the balloon within the urethra will cause trauma.

Drainage devices are usually composed of either a bag or valve devices. Bags are either discrete leg bags, which have a capacity of 500 ml, or large night bags, which are used overnight or in immobile patients and have a capacity range of 1,000–2,000 ml. A 'flip-flow' valve or tap device can be used to cycle the bladder, allowing the bladder to have a more normal voiding pattern that preserves muscle tone. Patients find these devices rather more convenient and discreet. They should be used in caution in patients with high pressure retention, acontractile bladder with diminished sensation or poorly compliant patients, as these patients must empty their bladders every 2–4 hours.

Male catheterisation

The urethra can be divided into to three segments for urethral catheterisation: the penile urethra, bulbo-membranous urethra (surrounded by sphincter), and prostatic urethra (Figure 20.1).

Understanding urethral anatomy is important because one can appreciate that the bend in the penile urethra can be straightened by stretching the penis perpendicularly to the body, facilitating the passage of the catheter. Local anaesthetic gel does not often make it around the bend to anaesthetise the membranous urethra. This can be a source of discomfort as the catheter is passed. Reassuring the patient and asking them to take slow deep breaths can help them relax, ensuring that the catheterisation is as atraumatic as possible. Furthermore, the prostate is located at the second bend of the 'S' and it is here that outlet obstruction is caused in men with urinary retention and makes catheterisation difficult.

If present, the foreskin should be retracted. Anaesthetic gel should be slowly inserted into the urethral meatus, and then ideally a penile clamp should be placed for 10 minutes. In practice, a clamp is rarely applied. The patient should be warned that introduction of the lignocaine gel into the urethra will result in 'stinging', which will settle as the anaesthetic takes effect.

Holding the penis up with one hand, the chosen catheter should be inserted with the other hand into the external meatus. It should be gently advanced without undue force. If resistance is met, forceful insertion must not be performed, but continuous gentle pressure should be applied, thereby trying to ascertain the level of obstruction.

Entry into the bladder will result in drainage of urine. If there is no drainage, gentle abdominal pressure to encourage urine flow may be used. Alternatively,

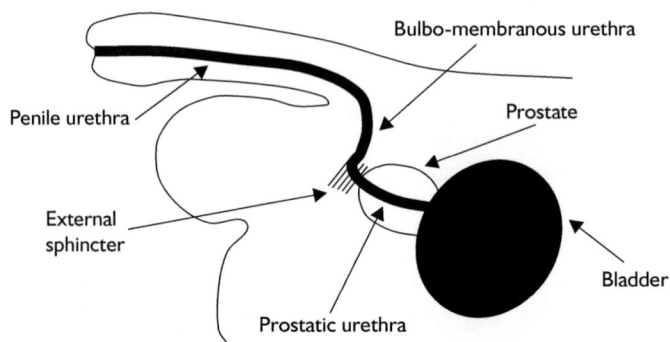

Figure 20.1 Male anatomy.

a 50 ml bladder syringe could be used to instil sterile water into the catheter and if the tip is in the bladder an equal amount will subsequently drain.

Having established the correct position of the catheter the balloon used to secure it should be gradually inflated with water for injection. The exact volume needed will depend on the type of catheter; generally 10 millilitres is standard. Saline should not be used for the balloon as it may erode the catheter material. Care should be taken when inflating the balloon, since inflation of the balloon within the urethra could result in severe trauma.

The catheter should be then attached to a fresh drainage bag or a valve device. Following catheterisation the foreskin must be replaced to avoid para-phimosis occurring. If catheterisation is performed for acute retention of urine then it is useful to record the immediate amount of urine drained, as this may help to determine subsequent investigations and treatment.

Difficult catheterisation – male

The inability of passage of the catheter past the bulbo-membranous urethral bend is commonly encountered and can be remedied through simple measures such as using double the amount of lubricating anaesthetic gel, which may prove useful in helping the catheter slip past the 'S' bend. A curved tip coudé catheter (Figure 20.2) is often used, which follows the natural curvature of the urethra into the bladder. This catheter may also be useful for patients having had a transurethral resection of prostate (TURP), where a lip can persist at the bladder neck.

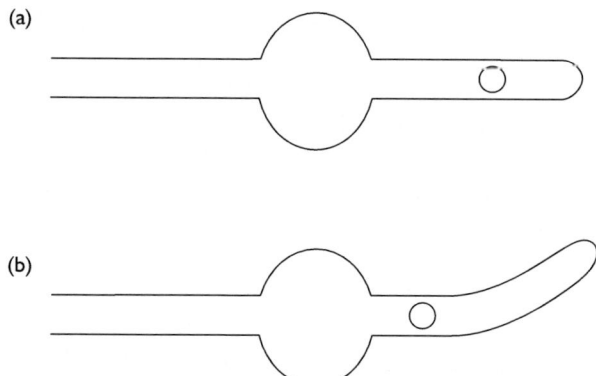

Figure 20.2 (a) Standard Foley catheter; (b) coudé tip catheter (note curve).

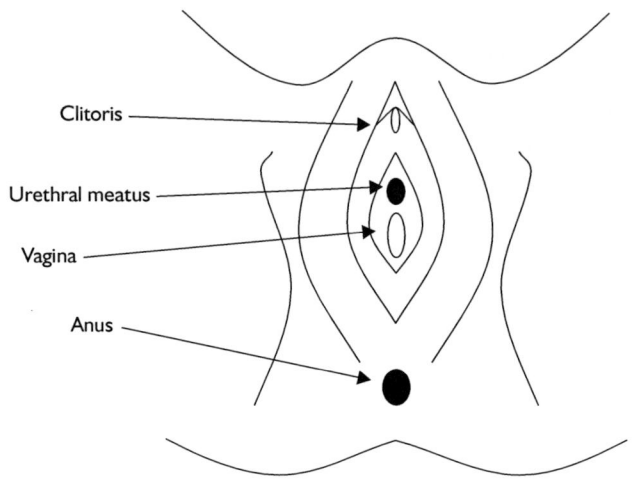

Figure 20.3 Female anatomy.

Female catheterisation

Correct identification of the urethral meatus is the most important factor in successful catheterisation in women (Figure 20.3). The female urethra is short at approximately 4 cm in length and is located anterior to the vagina. Occasionally it may be on the anterior vaginal wall and can only be felt as a depression in the vaginal mucosa. The clitoris is often confused with the urethral meatus, especially if the urethra is hidden on the anterior wall.

Shorter catheters are available for female patients and the same aseptic technique should be used for any catheterisation (see above). After positioning the patient in a 'frog-leg' position with the hips abducted, the genital area is prepared. The labia are then parted and the urethral meatus identified. Lubricating local anaesthetic gel is instilled into the urethra and the catheter gently inserted. There is no need to wait as long as with male catheterisation for the local anaesthetic to take effect, due to the short length of the urethra. The desired effect of the gel here is mainly lubrication. Once drainage of urine is established the balloon may be inflated and the catheter attached to the appropriate continence device.

Difficult catheterisation – female

This is uncommon and is generally related to obesity and inadequate positioning of the patient, making visualisation of the urethral meatus difficult. The use of a speculum may help, but ensuring that the patient is well positioned and having good lighting are more useful. If the meatus is on the anterior vaginal wall, a catheter can be directed anteriorly with a vaginally placed finger as a guide. Care should be taken when catheterising post-menopausal women who have reduced vaginal lubrication and/or atrophic vaginitis, which may make the procedure difficult.

Post-catheter documentation

It is an essential requirement that any invasive procedure is documented in the medical notes. Important information should include indication for insertion, date of insertion, type of catheter, residual urine, colour of urine drained, and difficulty of insertion.

Complications

Urethral catheterisation is a safe and generally well-tolerated procedure. However, complications may arise, some of which are detailed in Table 20.2 with suggested management and prevention plans.

Suprapubic catheterisation

Long-term urethral catheters should ideally be promptly replaced with a suprapubic catheter. Long-term urethral catheters are not advisable due to the urethral trauma they commonly inflict.

The suprapubic catheter should be sited by a urological surgeon, who may want to give a general anaesthetic so that the bladder can be distended, which facilitates the suprapubic puncture. Once the suprapubic tract has 'matured' (epithelialised), usually six to eight weeks post-puncture, the catheter may be changed for the first time. The first catheter change should ideally be performed under the care of a urology team; subsequent changes then at intervals of three months by district or practice nurses.

Table 20.2 Complications of urethral catheterisation.

Complication	Management/prevention
UTI	Treat infection only if symptomatic Colonisation does not necessitate antibiotics Increase fluid intake
Encrustation	Regular catheter changes 8 to 12 weeks at least; sooner if necessary Increase fluid intake
Blockages/bypassing	Regular catheter changes Bladder washouts Bladder instillation (e.g. Suby G) Increase fluid intake
Haematuria	Treat UTI Increase fluid intake Do not attribute to presence of catheter alone. Investigate upper and lower tracts with imaging and cystoscopy
Bladder spasm	Reduce balloon volume (reduces irritation of balloon on trigone) Anticholinergic medications (e.g. oxybutinin)
Traumatic displacement	Ensure catheter extruded intact Retained fragments can be nidus for stone formation
Paraphimosis	Ensure foreskin replaced after insertion/change of catheter
Acquired hypospadias	Caused by pressure necrosis of urethra by chronic usage Ensure catheter is not pulling Consider suprapubic catheter
Balloon unable to be deflated	Ensure always fill with water Cut valve to allow water to drain Consider USS guided puncture of balloon

Key points

- Indwelling catheters are safe and well tolerated.
- Good knowledge of male and female uro-genital anatomy is needed for trouble free catheterisation.
- Aseptic technique should be used at all times when catheterising patients.
- Catheter selection together with the appropriate continence device should be well considered according to the indications and patient needs.
- Regular follow-up and review of patients is needed by GPs and district/practice nurses to avoid any catheter related complications.

Further reading and bibliography

Kumar, P. and Pati, J. (2007) Urinary catheterisation. In: *Urological Emergencies in Hospital Medicine* (eds. I. S. Shergill, M. Arya, H. R. Patel and I. S. Gill), pp. 141–51. Quay Books, London.

CHAPTER 21

The nature and the role of the General Practitioner with a Specialist Interest (GPwSI)

Nitika Silhi and Aravinda Guniyangodage

What is a GPwSI?

There are currently more than 1,700 registered GPwSIs in the United Kingdom. The Department of Health defines a GPwSI as 'a General Practitioner (GP) with a specialist interest who supplements their core generalist role by delivering an additional high quality service to meet the needs of their patients. Working principally in the community they deliver a clinical service beyond the scope of their core professional role or may undertake advanced interventions not normally undertaken by their peers. They will have demonstrated appropriate skills and competencies to deliver those services without direct supervision'. Hence being a GPwSI is not about role substitution or cheap labour. It is about developing the NHS workforce and in particular the primary/secondary care interface and delivering care in the most appropriate way when and where necessary.

The origin of GPwSIs lies in the NHS Plan 2000, which envisaged 1,000 GPwSIs easing the burden on secondary care by offering more outpatient appointments and hence fewer secondary care referrals by 2006. This commitment was reinforced when in 2002 a further government document outlined plans for at least one million more outpatient appointments (around 10%) to take place in the community rather than the hospital, underlying the government's enthusiasm for more healthcare activity to take place in primary and community settings rather than in acute hospital trusts.

In 2006 urology was one of six specialities selected by the Department of Health to participate in a year long project entitled 'care closer to home' arguing that urology's increased medicalisation provided an ideal opportunity to start managing a growing urological workload in the community. Five urology demonstration sites were set up, yet only one site, in Bradford, directly involved GPs. The current top three GPwSI interests in England in order of popularity are Dermatology, Minor Surgery and Coronary Heart Disease. Similarly, since the advent of practice-based commissioning urology has fallen behind other surgical specialities, such as Ear, Nose and Throat and Orthopaedics. What has caused this lack of schemes? Certainly urology is a big money spinner for hospitals who would be reluctant to lose the income, but there are many other practical and professional factors such as skills and time that may also come into play.

Are GPwSIs needed?

There are many urological conditions suitable for management in the community, including lower urinary tract symptoms, erectile dysfunction, infertility and female urinary incontinence. In recent years, urology has become increasingly medicalised with the advent of effective pharmaceutical treatments for conditions such as benign prostatic hypertrophy and erectile dysfunction. Patient groups have been strong vocal advocates for GPwSI-led clinics. Patients are happier with local services nearer to their home and welcome the move into the community, as do cash-strapped Primary Care Trusts, who see this as possible savings. Patients experience shorter waiting times from referral to consultation; easy access for communication between physician and patient; reduced travelling time; familiar surroundings; and joint discussion of management and treatment among patient, GP and specialist. Managing more of these conditions in the community increases local capacity in urology and can enhance the quality and decrease the quantity of referrals made to consultant urologists. This means improved communication and relationships between the specialist and GP with better patient management and reduced specialist reattendances with increased patient follow-up by the GP. Ultimately, the GP referring to the GPwSI should see a reduction in the number of times the patient requests review and the secondary care specialist should see a reduction in hospital admissions. It empowers general practitioners, giving them more opportunities for training and education. However, one must bear in mind that the overriding need for a GPwSI-led service is to improve the care of patients suffering from urological pathology.

How to set up a GPwSI urology clinic in primary care

Prior to commencing the project there are three questions you should really ask yourself:

1. Do you have the time?
2. Do you have the energy?
3. Do you have the support of your colleagues/partners?

It is essential before you start to have a good plan of action with an idea of referral patterns and numbers as well as available financial resources. Then you will need to identify allies to support you in this endeavour, particularly an influential local consultant urologist with whom you can establish a good rapport as well as a supportive PCT. In order to convince others that this service will be necessary, one must gather evidence including numbers of patients seen with a urological condition in your practice, current outpatient waiting times to see a consultant urologist, local referral rates to secondary care and anecdotal reports from patients and patient groups who feel this service will be beneficial. Financially it is important to set tariffs based upon the National Tariff to calculate the income generated or savings that could be made. An easy exercise to undertake prior to starting would be to complete a SWOT analysis looking at the strengths, weaknesses, opportunities and threats of becoming a GPwSI and setting up a GPwSI clinic.

The next step would be to formulate a business plan and present it to either the Primary Care Trust (PCT) or your local commissioning cluster lead (Practice-Based Commissioning lead). This will provide direct answers regarding the funding of the clinic, the place where the service will be provided, the record systems used, the equipment needed and the administration support available.

The envisaged scope of the clinic may include a full diagnostic and management service, incorporating minor surgery or management of chronic conditions. One must be stringent in identifying those patients who would be more appropriately referred to secondary care and thus who are not suitable for attendance at a GPwSI clinic. We recommend that this triage of referrals is performed by the GPwSI themselves as it aids in maintaining good contacts with secondary care. One of the pitfalls of becoming a GPwSI is that many of your colleagues and peers may begin to see you as an expert in the field. It is important to realise your own limitations and remember that you are not a consultant but a GPwSI. It will also help foster relationships with secondary care consultants who may feel that GPwSI clinics will take away funding and destabilise their service. By ensuring that more serious and complex cases are seen in secondary care you are sending out a strong and vital message to both primary and secondary care colleagues.

Organisation should be a priority and no shortcuts should be taken as regards provision of secretarial and information technology support. Good and accurate record keeping is vital for clinical governance and medico-legal purposes and the GPwSI should ensure that all relevant correspondence is sent to the referring GP. Complaints should be handled in accordance with the PCT's complaints procedure.

It is always a good idea to keep an eye on further developments in the medico-political world, particularly with regard to the ongoing sustainability of the clinic. Once funding has been secured and the clinic is up and running it is essential to plan what would happen if you went on holiday or decided to leave. It is vital that the service is not dependent upon one person's knowledge or skill, for this might lead to its eventual downfall.

Obtaining the knowledge and recognised qualifications

First and foremost one must have an interest in the field (e.g. urology) or, during training, have had significant exposure to the specific speciality. Knowledge and clinical/practical skills can be gained via a variety of sources. A diploma in the speciality is recommended via attendance at a lecture-based course or via distance learning. Sitting in on a minimum number of supervised clinics in secondary care will help consolidate the theory learnt. Any practical procedures performed should initially be supervised prior to independent practice. A logbook documenting these is mandatory.

Local PCTs may have their own requirements for GPwSIs in each speciality, but it is wiser to follow the national accreditation system for GPwSIs if there is one. The RCGP have published guidelines on the DoH website for several specialities (unfortunately not for urology as yet). These include a requirement for the GPwSI to have one clinic a month with a consultant who acts as a mentor.

A GPwSI is fully responsible for the clinical service that they provide and as such it would be a prudent move to inform your defence organisation of your involvement as a GPwSI. In some cases if you are directly employed by the hospital trust you may be covered by their indemnity scheme. However, if you are employed as an independent provider then you may have to boost your level of insurance.

Once established and practising as a GPwSI one should continue to work closely with the consultant, having frequent joint case discussions and regular audit. It is essential to continue with professional development by attending further courses and seminars and perusal of the relevant literature, and in fact the RCGP has recommended that GPwSIs attend at least 15 hours a year of lectures for continued professional development. It is important that all of this is documented in the GPwSI's personal development portfolio, as this can be used as part of the annual appraisal. It is important to note that a GPwSI does not require a separate appraisal as a GP and as a GPwSI. Another form of ensuring that the GPwSI is up to date is to become a member of the relevant postgraduate speciality organisation, e.g. the British Association of Urological Surgeons.

Why be a GPwSI?

A major reason for becoming a GPwSI is to provide a higher level of care to patients and by doing so gain personal satisfaction. By participating in clinical care outside general practice a GP is likely to have better self-esteem due to the additional interest and personal development offered. This in turn may lead to enhanced retention of GPs and delayed burnout. Working in conjunction with secondary care consultants will help break down barriers, increase effective communication and improve continuity of patient care. This enhanced teamworking could also apply between local GPs. For the patient, GPwSI clinics usually represent improved patient access, reduced waiting times, flexibility and a less intimidating, more personal service with similar clinical outcomes to those in secondary care.

It is unlikely, as previously thought, that GPwSI clinics will reduce demand. Rather, as is the case in much of the NHS, the clinic is likely to meet a currently unmet need. It was thought that the clinics would reduce hospital waiting lists with a monetary saving to the PCT. However, recent reports including one from the Audit Commission show some GPwSI services are likely to be more expensive than hospital care and may not cut waiting times or be more convenient for patients. It is also important to ensure that the GPwSI clinic does not become a second class service by lowering clinical standards and denying patients access to the right service. It is important for GPwSIs to ensure that they have appropriate training, accreditation and specialist support to guarantee quality and safety. One of the major arguments against GPwSI is that their creation will downgrade and fragment general practice leading to the devaluation and loss of generalism as a speciality. However, those who work as GPwSIs deny that they value their specialist role more and even report that it has invigorated their punctured enthusiasm.

Conclusion

The government is committed to delivering more healthcare in the community, but is less certain when it comes to deciding by whom this care will be provided. It could be that secondary care consultants may deliver the care in a primary care setting, in which case there will be less of a requirement for GPwSIs. The original model, however, envisaged specialist generalists working independently of consultants in the community. The only thing that remains clear about the future is that there will be an intermediate tier of healthcare between primary and secondary care manned by sub-specialists such as GPs, pharmacists or consultants. It is anticipated that the service they provide will play a vital role in the transfer of secondary care into the community, be it through practice-based commissioning or a more central governmental funding mechanism.

Key points

- Be determined – nothing ever changes in the NHS without a fight!
- Do your research and have a good plan of action with an idea of referral patterns and numbers as well as available financial resources.
- Write everything down – from business plans to personal development plans.
- Ensure a good working relationship with the secondary care consultant.
- It is important for GPwSIs to ensure that they have appropriate training, qualifications, accreditation and specialist support to guarantee quality and safety.
- Keep your wits about you!

Further reading and bibliography

General practitioners with special interests, January 2006, RCGP information sheet. http://www.rcgp.org.uk/pdf/ISS_INFO_11_JAN06.pdf; accessed June 2008.
GPs with special interests (GPwSIs). http://www.bma.org.uk/ap.nsf/Content/GPsWI; accessed June 2008.

CHAPTER 22

Imaging techniques in urology

Christopher Blick, Miles Walkden, Nilay Patel and Asif Muneer

Introduction

Diagnostic imaging in urology has undergone significant developments in recent years. The imaging modalities now available can provide high-resolution anatomical images of both normal and pathological tissue. This has been facilitated by the availability of sophisticated post-processing software which allows greater resolution and also three-dimensional reconstruction. The basic principles of the more commonly utilised modalities in urology will be outlined, together with the uses of the technique in secondary care.

Plain X-ray and intravenous urography (IVU)

A two-dimensional plain X-ray incorporating the kidneys, ureter and bladder (KUB) has traditionally been utilised to assess patients with suspected renal colic. The presence of an opacity in the renal tract requires further confirmation with either an IVU or CT scan. The IVU involves taking a series of plain films after the administration of intravenous contrast. Although commonly performed as a first line investigation in patients with renal colic, this has gradually been replaced by non-contrast CT scans. Following the control film (which is a KUB) and administration of intravenous contrast, the IVU has a nephrogram phase whereby contrast is filtered into the proximal convoluted tubule. This is followed by the pyelogram phase whereby the contrast is concentrated as it passes through the renal tubule. IVU can be performed to image the collecting system as part of the assessment of haematuria when the

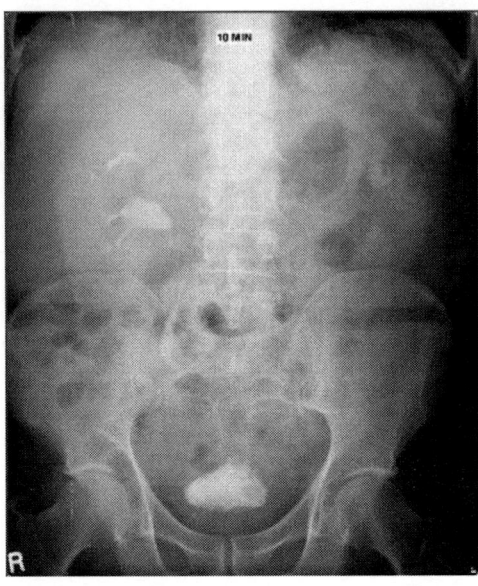

Figure 22.1 IVU demonstrating a bladder mass with obstruction of the left kidney. The bladder tumour was resected and was found to be invasive.

ultrasound scan and cystoscopy reveal no lesion. It is also useful in the post-operative follow up of ureteric surgery, e.g. post-stricture surgery. Figure 22.1 shows an IVU obtained from a patient diagnosed with a bladder lesion. One of the main complications of IVU can result from the use of contrast agents and ensuing contrast reactions – these are discussed in Chapter 7.

Ultrasonography

Ultrasound is a non-invasive, painless imaging technique which is widely available, low cost and easy to use. There is no radiation exposure, there are no known harmful effects of standard ultrasound imaging and real-time images are generated.

The ultrasound probe houses a transducer generating high-frequency sound waves (typically 2–18 MHz) and a receiver detecting sound waves reflected from tissues. The variation in the density of tissue boundaries determines the echogenicity of the tissue and hence the reflection of the sound waves.

Kidneys ultrasound

Ultrasound is the initial imaging modality of choice in any patient with an unexplained elevation of the serum creatinine level or recent onset of renal dysfunction. In most instances, ultrasound images in the setting of acute renal failure are normal, but ultrasound can detect hydronephrosis/hydroureter which occurs in post renal obstruction. The size of the kidney and ureter on ultrasound may aid in diagnosing the aetiology of hydronephrosis (i.e. obstruction secondary to ureteropelvic junction obstruction or stones) as opposed to non-obstructive dilatation secondary to vesicoureteric reflux.

Ultrasound has limited use in the diagnosis of acute pyelonephritis, although it is useful to exclude coexisting abnormalities such as stones, cysts or congenital abnormalities. Ultrasound can be used to detect and monitor the progress of complications of pyelonephritis, such as renal abscesses or pyonephrosis.

Ultrasound will detect large renal tumours appearing as heterogenous echogenic masses (Figure 22.2) and is the modality of choice when imaging renal cysts. Diagnosis of a cyst based on ultrasound findings is 95–98% accurate. Sonography alone cannot distinguish between benign and malignant cysts, but the use of the Bosniak classification can help categorise the probability of malignancy.

Bladder ultrasound

Ultrasound is used to measure bladder volume and post-void residual urine volumes. It is also used to identify masses within the bladder which can be

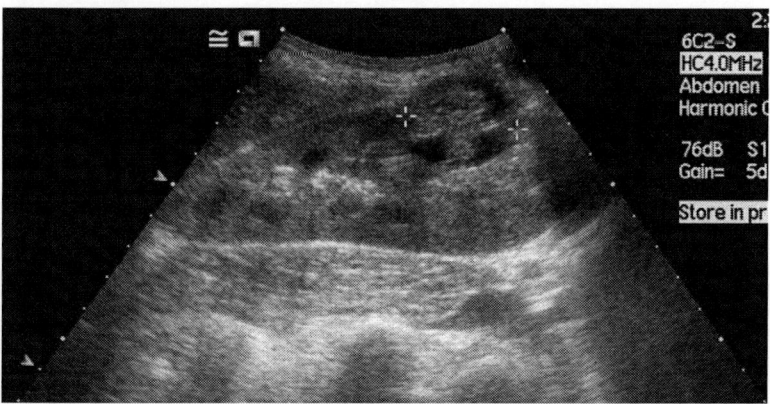

Figure 22.2 Renal neoplasm detected on ultrasound as part of the investigation for haematuria. The patient underwent a CT scan for further staging.

diagnosed with relative certainty if the bladder is full. The appearance of transitional cell carcinoma (TCC) within the bladder is indistinguishable sonographically from other neoplasms. Carcinoma *in situ* and squamous metaplasia are generally undetectable by ultrasound but may be seen as focal bladder wall thickening.

Prostate ultrasound

Originally hailed as a possible diagnostic modality for prostate cancer, transrectal ultrasound is now mainly used as a guiding tool for prostate biopsies and the determination of prostate volume prior to planning surgery or radiation therapy. Transrectal ultrasound is also used in the evaluation of the infertile male particularly those men with azoospermia and a low volume ejaculate (< 1.5 ml). It is used to investigate obstructive causes of azoospermia by looking for cystic dilation of the ejaculatory ducts and seminal vesicles.

Urethral ultrasound

Sonourethrography has been shown to be accurate, sensitive, and specific for the diagnosis and assessment of penile and bulbar urethral strictures. However, the applicability of urethral ultrasound has evolved to include planning for surgical approach to urethral stricture disease.

Scrotal ultrasound

Ultrasound has long been the standard for the imaging evaluation of scrotal masses, with a sensitivity of nearly 100%. However, no reliable sonographic criteria are available to distinguish a malignant lesion from a focal benign intratesticular lesion, such as infarction, haemorrhage, infection, or non-germ-cell tumour. The common scrotal conditions presenting to primary care physicians include:

- **Hydrocoele**: sonographic inspection of a hydrocoele must include careful imaging of the testicle, particularly because the hydrocoele occasionally renders the testis impalpable and therefore may conceal a testicular mass.
- **Varicocoele**: sonography can be beneficial in the case of subclinical varicocoeles, for which the physical examination findings are normal but the

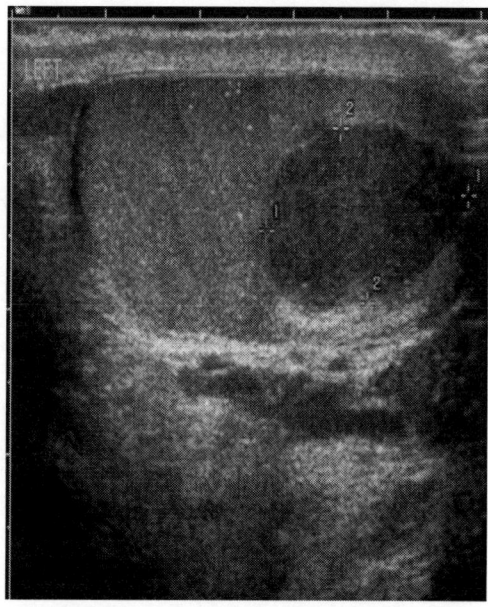

Figure 22.3 Testicular seminoma detected by ultrasonography conducted on the same day as the referral. Tumour markers were normal and the patient underwent a radical orchidectomy.

patient has infertility, scrotal pain, or other symptoms suggesting a varicocoele. The acute onset of a varicocoele, particularly on the left side should have combined imaging of the kidneys to exclude a synchronous renal mass.

- **Infection of epididymis/testis**: this is characterised by focal, peripheral, hypoechoic testicular lesions that are poorly defined, amorphous or crescent-shaped. There may be associated testicular/epididymal hyperaemia and a reactive hydrocoele.

- **Testicular trauma**: ultrasound is the imaging method of choice for scrotal trauma. Sonography helps to evaluate testicular rupture as an adjunct to the clinical history and examination. Testicular rupture is seen as focal alterations of testicular echogenicity correlating with areas of intratesticular haemorrhage or infarction.

- **Scrotal lumps**: ultrasound is useful in the assessment of scrotal masses and allows the differentiation of benign lesions such as epididymal cysts from malignant lesions in the testicle which appear as solid, echo poor lesions with an abnormal architecture (Figure 22.3).

Nuclear medicine

In nuclear medicine, the patient is given a radioactive tracer agent either by mouth, intravenous injection or inhalation. The tracer goes to the target organ and can then be imaged with a gamma camera, a positron emission tomography (PET) scanner or a probe; these record the radiation photons emitted by the radioactive tracer which are converted into images of the target organs. Nuclear medicine can often yield more information than other imaging techniques and is less invasive than exploratory surgery. They involve limited radiation, are relatively pain free and as a general rule allergic reactions to radionuclide tracer agents do not occur. Nuclear medicine is, however, time-consuming and requires the patient to remain motionless to obtain optimal images.

DMSA scans (cortical scintigraphy)

This test involves the use of ^{99m}Tc dimercaptosuccinic acid (DMSA). This provides imaging of the renal parenchyma. Decreased uptake occurs with renal masses, scar tissue, pyelonephritis and obstruction. A DMSA scan can also be used to assess split function, renal ectopia, infarction, acute renal failure and renal vascular thrombosis.

An obstructed kidney will usually appear large with reduced uptake. Cortical scintigraphy allows monitoring of scar formation from recurrent urinary tract infections and VUR. This can be helpful in determining the necessity for and timing of surgical intervention particularly in paediatric cases.

Dynamic renal scintigraphy

Renal scintigraphy is a very sensitive modality for the evaluation of renal blood flow and renal function. Diuretic renography is used to help differentiate non obstructive dilatation of the pelvicalyceal systems from obstruction. The current agent of choice for dynamic renal scintigraphy is ^{99m}Tc-MAG3 (mercaptoacetyltriglycine). Indications for dynamic renal scintigraphy include (1) evaluating obstruction, (2) monitoring patients with medical renal disease, (3) monitoring patients with neurogenic bladder dysfunction, (4) diagnosing renovascular hypertension, (5) assessing post-operative results, (6) evaluating donors and recipients of renal transplants, and (7) determining relative (split)

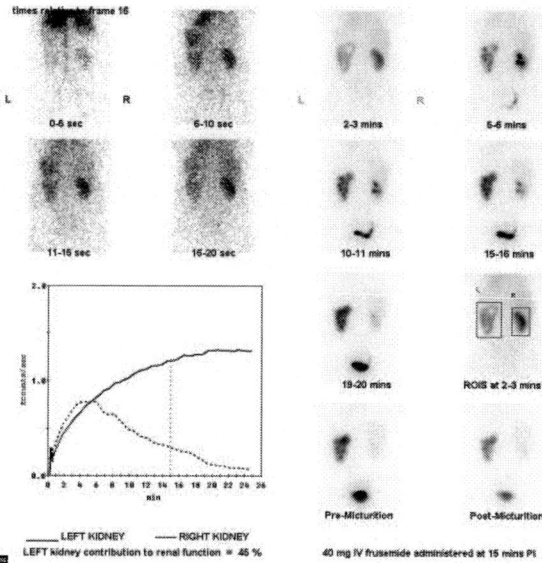

Figure 22.4 MAG 3 renogram illustrating obstruction of the left kidney. The is no excretion of radionuclide despite the administration of furosemide at 15 minutes. The left kidney is contributing 45% function and therefore underwent a pyeloplasty.

renal function. Following the perfusion phase of the examination and once the isotope has accumulated in the renal pelvis a prompt washout of the isotope occurs through the ureters and into the bladder, producing a characteristic curve. In non-obstructed but dilated collecting systems, differentiation from obstruction is aided by the administration of intravenous furosemide administration. The retention of the radiopharmaceutical in the renal pelvis despite furosemide injection is indicative of obstruction (Figure 22.4).

Radionuclide cystography

This technique is useful in the assessment of vesicoureteric reflux (VUR). There are two techniques described:

- **Direct voiding cystourethrography**. The bladder is filled with a technetium-labelled compound and a gamma camera is placed underneath the patient. Reflux is then identified from the serial images. However, routine cystography with radiography contrast is superior for the initial study because it helps assess for VUR and helps determine the grade of VUR, which is not possible with the nuclear cystogram.

- **Indirect voiding cystourethrography** involves intravenous radionuclide administration and hence eliminates catheterisation in young children. The disadvantages are that the bladder is not sufficiently distended, which may reduce the chance of reflux, and residual activity in the kidney may mask small amounts of reflux. This study can be used in the initial diagnosis of VUR or to evaluate patients with urinary tract infections. Nuclear cystography is best for follow-up of known reflux, post-operative assessment of antireflux surgery, or evaluation of siblings of index children with VUR because the presence of reflux is the primary endpoint in these situations and nuclear cystography exposes children to much less radiation.

Bone scintigraphy

Bone scintigraphic agents have historically included a variety of ^{99m}Tc-labelled phosphate and diphosphonate compounds, of which methylene diphosphonate and hydroxy methylene diphosphonate are currently used. Similar to the early agent pyrophosphate (still used for myocardial infarct imaging), these radiopharmaceuticals tend to localise in areas of dystrophic calcification or necrotic tissues. Metastatic prostate lesions are typically located in the axial skeleton

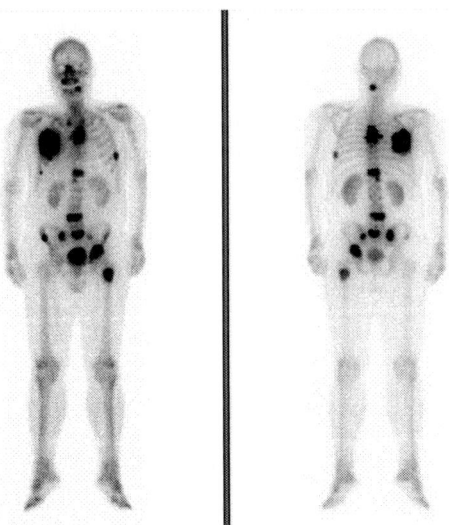

Figure 22.5 A patient with newly diagnosed prostate cancer undergoing a bone scan demonstrating multiple lesions indicative of metastatic disease.

(Figure 22.5). Degenerative disease is commonly seen as increased uptake in the periphery of the bone, whereas metastatic lesions are located more centrally.

Computed tomography (CT)

A CT scanner uses an X-ray tube sited opposite a detector. The most recent generation of scanners, termed 'spiral' or 'helical', allow rapid scanning of patients and therefore eliminate movement artefacts. The scanner generates a series of pixels which is dependent on the tissue density, following which a computer calculates the attenuation value of each pixel and reconstructs this into an image. In order to allow differentiation of adjacent organs, oral or intravenous contrast is utilised (for contrast reactions see Chapter 7). The data can be formatted to allow images to be viewed in two or three dimensions. CT is useful in the investigation of renal and bladder lesions and the staging of neoplasms (Figure 22.6). Non-contrast CT scans of the urinary tract are gradually replacing the IVU examination in the assessment of renal colic as the sensitivity approaches 100% with CT (c.f. sensitivity of 50–60% with IVU) and also allows the detection of other pathology together with avoiding the use of intravenous contrast (Figure 22.7).

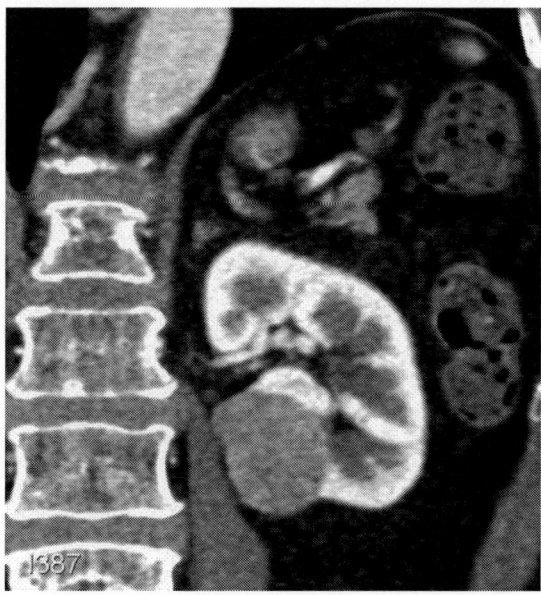

Figure 22.6 Contrast CT scan showing a lower pole renal lesion of the left kidney.

227

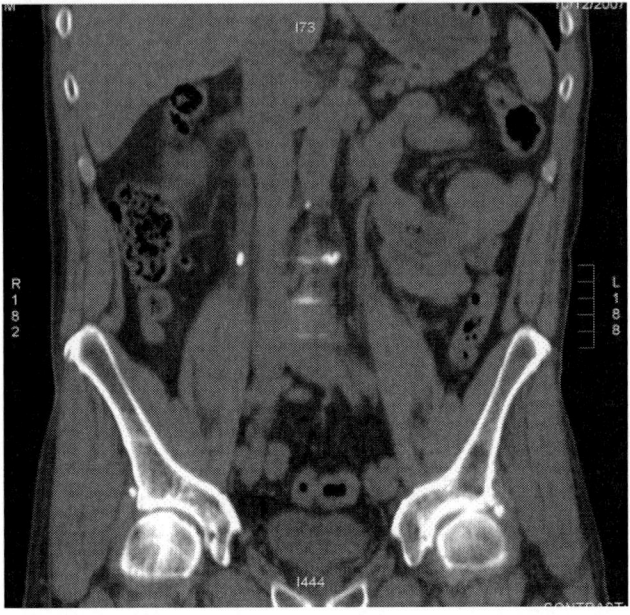

Figure 22.7 Acute non-contrast CT scan showing a right ureteric stone.

Magnetic resonance imaging (MRI)

MRI combines a strong magnetic field together with radiofrequency (RF) energy to study the behaviour and distribution of protons in fat and water. The physics of MRI is extremely complex and is only briefly discussed. Once a patient is placed in the scanner, the protons in the patient's tissues align themselves along the direction of the magnetic field. A radiofrequency pulse is applied, which results in deflection of the protons off their axis along the magnetic field. When the protons realign themselves with the magnetic field, a signal is produced which is detected by an antenna. With the help of computer analysis the signals are converted into an image.

The process by which the protons realign themselves with the magnetic field is referred to as relaxation and is subdivided into T1 and T2. Different tissues undergo different rates of relaxation. Care must be exercised in patients with embedded ferromagnetic objects (e.g. shrapnel) and in those with implants (e.g. pacemaker wires). In addition to this, MRI should not be performed on patients with cardiac pacemakers or aneurysm clips. The use of MRI in urological practice includes cross-sectional imaging of renal and bladder neoplasms, assessment of prostate cancer, imaging of penile cancer and MR urography.

Interventional techniques

Interventional techniques utilise real-time ultrasound scanning or CT. Commonly performed techniques under local anaesthetic include percutaneous insertion of nephrostomy tubes to relieve obstructed collecting systems and CT or ultrasound guided biopsy of lesions. Fluoroscopy is used to insert antegrade ureteric stents via nephrostomy tracks and also to perform retrograde pyelography as part of the assessment for haematuria.

Index

acute pyelonephritis 34, 41–2
allergy 78
analgesia 71
androgen ablation 157
angiokeratoma 82
antibiotics 39–40, 182
artificial urethral sphincter 51
asthenozoospermia 28
azoospermia 26–7
  investigation 28–9
  management 29–30
  non-obstructive 27
  obstructive 26–7

bacterial persistence 35
bacteriuria 33, 35
bag specimen of urine 180
balanitis xerotica obliterans 79–80, 168, 170–1
balanoposthitis 87–8, 168, 171–2
Behcet disease 81
benign conditions 95
  scrotum and testis 57–65
benign prostatic hyperplasia 91–8
  surgery 97–8
  treatment 96–8
biofeedback 50
bisphosphonates 161
bladder cancer 111–20
  advanced 113–14
  diagnosis 115–16
  discussion with patient 117–18
  examination 114
  haematuria 113
  high grade 119

incidence 111
lower urinary tract symptoms 113
management 114, 118
muscle-invasive 119–20
risk factors 112–13
staging 116–17
superficial 118–19
treatment 116–17
types 112
bladder diary 48
bladder outlet obstruction 95
  treatment 96–9
bladder training 51
bone scintigraphy 226–7
BOO see bladder outlet obstruction
Bowen's disease 83
Bowenoid papulosis 83–4
brachytherapy 149–50
BSU see bag specimen of urine
Burch colposuspension 51
BXO see balanitis xerotica obliterans

calculi 67–75
  spontaneous passage 73
candidiasis 85
catheterisation see urethral catheterisation
catheters 204–5
CBAVD see congenital bilateral absence of vas
CHD see coronary heart disease
chemotherapy 160
circinate balanitis 81
circumcision 81, 167
  contraindications 174–5

legal issues   175
non-medical reasons   172, 175
sexually transmitted diseases   172–3
squamous cell carcinoma   172
surgical complications   174
surgical technique   173–4
urinary tract infection and   172
clam cystoplasty   54
clotting screen   106
computed tomography   227
computerised tomography scan   107–8
congenital bilateral absence of vas   26, 29
cord compression   156
coronary heart disease
erectile dysfunction and   6
cortical scintigraphy   224
cranberry juice   40
cryptorchidism   193–8
causes   194
complications   194
examination   195–6
history   195
investigation   196–7
management   197–9
surgery   197–9
CT-KUB *see* unenhanced helical computed tomography
cystitis   34, 178
cystoscopy   108, 116

detrusor injections   52
digital rectal examination   92
dipstix test   37–8, 47
DMSA scan   224
drainage devices   205
dynamic renal scintigraphy   224–5
dysfunctional voiding   187, 190
dysuria   104

eczema   78
ED *see* erectile dysfunction
ejaculatory duct obstruction   26
endocrine abnormalities   27
epididymal cysts   60–1
epididymal obstruction   26
epididymis   21, 58

imaging   223
epididymitis   62–3
erectile dysfunction   3–13
coronary heart disease and   6–7
definition   4
drugs and   9
first line treatments   10–11
history   5
hormone treatment   8
lifestyle changes   8
management   6–7
NHS treatment   9–10
PDE5 inhibitors   10–11
physical examination   5
psychosexual counselling   9
risk factors   4
second line treatments   11–12
specialist investigations   7
treatment   8–9
vacuum devices   11–12
erythrasma   85–6
erythroplasia of Queyrat   82–3
Escherichia coli   35, 40
ESWL *see* extra-corporeal shock wave lithotripsy
external beam radiotherapy   157
extra-corporeal shock wave lithotripsy   73

fixed drug eruption   78–9
foreskin   167–76
anatomy and development   168–9
examination   169
non-retractile   167–8
retractile incidence   169

General Practitioner with a Specialist Interest   213–18
benefits   214
description   213–14
need for   214
qualifications   216–17
reasons for becoming   217
record keeping   216
referral   215
setting up a clinic   215–16
urology   214

working with consultants 216–17
genetic abnormalities 27
germinal aplasia 27
giggle incontinence 187, 191
gland of Fordyce 82
Gleason grading system 144
GPwSI *see* General Practitioner with a
    Specialist Interest

haematuria 101–9
  assessment of urea and
    electrolytes 106
  bladder cancer 113
  causes 102–3
  classification 102–3
  evaluation of patients 103
  examination 105
  history 103–4
  investigations 105–8
  management 108–9
  prevalence 101–2
herpes simplex 86
high-intensity focused ultrasound 152–
  3
hormone deficiency 8–9
HSV *see* herpes simplex
hydrocoele 16
  clinical features 60
  idiopathic 59–60
  imaging 222
  treatment 60

ICSI *see* intracytoplasmic sperm
    injection
imaging techniques 219–29
  interventional 229
incontinence *see* urinary incontinence
infertility
  definition 25
  examination 27
  history 25–6
  investigations 28
  male 25–31
  referral to secondary care 31
  sexual history 26
intensity-modulated radiotherapy 148
intermittent hormone therapy 158

International Index of Erectile
    Function 5
International Prostate Symptom
    Score 92–3, 95
  low 96
  moderate to severe 96–7
intracytoplasmic sperm injection 30
intravenous urography 70, 107, 219–20
in vitro fertilisation 30
iodine 125 seeds 150
IPSS *see* International Prostate Symptom
    Score
iridium 192 rods 150
IVF *see in vitro* fertilisation
IVU *see* intravenous urography

Kaposi's sarcoma 84
kidney-ureter-bladder radiograph 70
KUB *see* kidney-ureter-bladder
    radiograph

lazy bladder 187
Levitra 4, 10
lichen planus 80
lichen sclerosus 79–80
lichen simplex 78
lifestyle changes 51
lower urinary tract symptoms 45
  assessment 92
  benign prostatic hyperplasia 91–8
  bladder cancer 113
  definitions 46
  examination 92–5
  history 92
  investigations 94
LS *see* lichen sclerosus
luteinising hormone releasing
    hormone 148, 157, 159
LUTS *see* lower urinary tract symptoms

magnetic resonance imaging 108, 228
maturation arrest 27
MESA *see* micro-epididymal sperm
    aspiration
micro-epididymal sperm aspiration 30
microscopy 38
midstream urine test 37–8, 47

mixed urinary incontinence   44
molluscum contagiosum   88
monosymptomatic nocturnal
        enuresis   189–90
morning serum testosterone   3, 6
Mullerian duct cyst   29

nocturnal polyuria   95
nuclear medicine   224

OATS syndrome   28
oestrogens   160
oligospermia   29
oligozoospermia   28
oral pharmacotherapy   50, 52–3
orchidopexy   25, 26
orchitis   62–3
overactive bladder syndrome   44
oxybutynin   52

pad testing   48
Paget's disease   84
patent processus vaginalis   195
PCB *see* plasma cell balanitis
PDE5 inhibitors   10–11
  safety   11–12
pearly penile papules   82
pelvic floor muscles   47, 50
penile prosthesis   12–13
percutaneous epididymal sperm
        aspiration   30
PESA *see* percutaneous epididymal
        sperm aspiration
phimosis   169–72
  management   171
  surgery   171–2
physiotherapy   50
plasma cell balanitis   80–1
post-void residual volume urine
        volume   94
prepuce *see* foreskin
prophylactic antibiotic therapy   35
prostate cancer   155–62
    active surveillance   138, 150–1
    advanced   157–8
    androgen ablation   157–9
    bisphosphonates   161

brachytherapy   149–50
chemotherapy   160
examination   156
grading   144
high-intensity focused
        ultrasound   152–3
history   141–2, 155
intermittent hormone therapy   158
investigations   156
localised   141–53
locally advanced   157
management   137–9, 143–4, 156
maximum androgen blockade   159–60
metatstatic   159–61
PSA and   133–4
radical prostatectomy   146–7, 158
radiotherapy   148–9, 157, 160–1
screening   133–4
staging   137–8
TNM classification   142
treatment   145–53
vasectomy and   22
prostate specific antigen   6, 131–9
    age-related   135–6
    density   136
    elevated levels   132
    examination   142–3
    following cancer treatment   138–9
    hormonal manipulation   139
    investigations   143
    isoforms   137
    prostate cancer and   132
    role   131
    specificity   135
    velocity   136–7
PSA *see* prostate specific antigen
psoriasis   77
psychosexual counselling   9
pubic lice   84–5
PVR *see* post-void residual volume urine
        volume
pyelonephritis   178
pyuria   35, 37

radical prostatectomy   158
radionuclide cystography   225–6
radiotherapy   160–1

Reiter's syndrome   81
renal colic *see* ureteric colic

sacral neuromodulation   54
scrotal conditions
  differential diagnosis   59
  examination   58
  history   58
  investigations   59
scrotum   57–8
  imaging   223
semen analysis, normal range   28
Sertoli cell only syndrome   29
sexually transmitted infections   26
sildenafil   10
skin disorders   77–88
  benign   77–82
  infections   84–8
  pre-malignant conditions   82–4
Solifenacin   52
spermatocoele *see* epididymal cysts
sperm granuloma   20
sperm retrieval   30
squamous cell carcinomas   172–3
steroids   160
stress incontinence   44, 187
  management   49–51
stress test   47
suprapubic catheterisation   209
syphilis   87

tadalafil   10
tamsulosin   72
tension-free vaginal tape   51
teratozoospermia   28
TESE *see* testicular exploration and
    sperm extraction
testes   57–8
  imaging   223
  lumps   58
  torsion   63–5
testicular cancer   121–8
  cryptorchidism and   194
  examination   123
  history   123
  incidence   122
  investigations   123–4

management   126–8
nonseminatomous germ cell
    tumours   126–8
prognosis   128
risk factors   123
Royal Marsden Hospital Staging
    System   124
seminomas   126–7
TNM staging system   125
types   122
testicular exploration and sperm
    extraction   30
testicular torsion   63–5
  clinical features   64
  differential diagnosis   64
  treatment   64–5
testicular volume   27
testosterone   159
tinea cruris   85
torted testicular appendages   65
transobturator tape   51
transurethral resection of prostate   207
transurethral resection of the
    prostate   98
TURP *see* transurethral resection of the
    prostate
Tyson's gland   82

ultrasonography   107, 220–3
  bladder   221–2
  kidneys   221
  prostate   222
  scrotum   222–3
  urethra   222
undescended testis *see* cryptorchidism
unenhanced helical computed
    tomography   70–1
ureter anatomy   69
ureteric colic   67–75
  dietary modification   74–5
  examination   69–70
  history   68
  incidence   68
  investigations   70–1
  management   71–2
  prevention   74–5
  referral   72

treatment   73
ureteroscopy   73
urethral anatomy
  male   206
urethral catheterisation   203–9
  complications   209–10
  consent   204
  difficult   207–9
  documentation   209
  female   208–9
  indications   203–4
  male   206–7
  patient preparation   204
urge incontinence   44, 187
  management   49, 51–4
urgency   44
urinalysis   70, 105–6, 180–1
urinary diversion   54
urinary incontinence
  aetiology   186
  assessment   45
  causes   45, 186–7
  children   185–91
  daytime   186–7, 190–1
  definition   43–4
  examination   46–7, 188
  history   45–6, 187–8
  investigations   47–8, 188–9
  management   49–54, 189–91
  nocturnal   186
  referral   48–9
  women   43–55
urinary markers   107
urinary tract imaging   107–8
urinary tract infection
  adults   33–42
  children   177–84
  classification   178
  complicated   34
  definitions   34–5
  epidemiology   33
  examination   36, 179
  history   36, 178–9
  incidence   33, 177
  investigations   36–9, 180–2
  isolated   34
  management   39–42, 182–3

microbiology   35
post-menopause   41
pregnancy   41
prognosis   183–4
radiological investigations   181–2
recurrent   34–5, 39–40
routes   35–6
uncomplicated   34
unresolved   34
urine storage   91
urine collection   36–7, 179–80
urine culture   38
urine cytology   48, 106–7
UTI *see* urinary tract infection

vacuum devices   11–12
vardenafil   10
varicocoele   16, 26, 30, 61–2
  associations   62
  clinical features   61
  grading   61
  imaging   222
  treatment   62
vas deferens obstruction   26
vasectomy   15–22
  antisperm antibodies   22
  complications   20–3
  counselling   17–18
  epididymectomy   21
  examination   16
  haematoma   20
  history   15–16
  incisional technique   18
  management   17–18
  no-scalpel technique   18
  operative technique   18–19
  post-operative care   19–20
  prostate cancer   22
  recanalisation   17
  reversal   17, 21–2
  scrotal pain   17, 21–2
  semen analysis   20
  spermatic cord denervation   21
  sperm granuloma   20
  vasal occlusion technique   19
vesico-ureteric reflux   183
Viagra   3, 10

voiding postponement   187
VUR *see* vesico-ureteric reflux

X-ray   219–20

Zoon's balanitis   80–1